RETINITIS PIGMENTOSA
Clinical Implications
of Current Research

ADVANCES IN EXPERIMENTAL MEDICINE AND BIOLOGY

Recent Volumes in this Series

To Werner K. Noell, M.D.,
whose work, almost ignored at first,
points the way to the future.

Foreword

The ARVO sectional meetings offer the opportunity to hold a symposium on some specialized subject. We have selected *retinitis pigmentosa* because it is a common disease and because current research holds an apparent promise for a future clinical resolution of this disease. Retinitis pigmentosa is a complicated condition. We may find that it is not a single disease, but possibly several diseases. Hopefully, anything we learn from our current research can be applied to the clinical aspects, in order that we may cure or at least gain a better understanding of the condition.

I want to call your attention to the word "symposium." Symposium is from the Greek, which means "drinking party." Its earliest use was from one of Socrates' students, who said that when Socrates attended a symposium, he usually stayed all night. The meaning of the word either degenerated or at least evolved, in the 16th century, as a meeting of a congenial and convivial group to discuss topics of their mutual interest. It later developed, in the early 1700's to a meeting whereby problems and investigative subjects could be discussed. I will leave it up to you as to whether this meeting indicates progress or deterioration of the definition of symposium.

The following book is a record of our symposium. In addition, we have included some of the material presented in other parts of the same meeting.

The smooth performance of this meeting was in large part due to the help of Ms. Joan Friedlein. The publication of this book would not have been possible without the tireless effort and skill of Mrs. Nancy Miller. A grant from the National Research Institute for Blindness, Incorporated was of great assistance in defraying the costs of the special speakers at the symposium.

Joseph A. C. Wadsworth

Duke University Eye Center
Durham, North Carolina

Contents

Contributors

WERNER ADRIAN, Lighttechnical Institute, University of Karlsruhe, Karlsruhe, West Germany

DANIEL M. ALBERT, Department of Ophthalmology and Visual Science, Yale University School of Medicine, 333 Cedar Street, New Haven, Connecticut 06510

W. BANKS ANDERSON, JR., Duke University Eye Center, Durham, North Carolina 27710

THOMAS S. BALDWIN, University of North Carolina School of Social Work, Chapel Hill, North Carolina 27514

JAMES BASTEK, Department of Ophthalmology, New Jersey Medical School (CMDNJ), Newark, New Jersey 07103

DONALD R. BERGSMA, Clinical Branch, National Eye Institute, National Institutes of Health, Bethesda, Maryland 20014

JOHN BOGDEN, Department of Preventive Medicine, New Jersey Medical School (CMDNJ), Newark, New Jersey 07103

NED BUYUKMIHCI, Department of Ophthalmology and Visual Science, Yale University School of Medicine, 333 Cedar Street, New Haven, Connecticut 06510

JAMES CHARLES, Department of Ophthalmology, New Jersey Medical School (CMDNJ), Newark, New Jersey 07103

ALFONSE CINOTTI, Department of Ophthalmology, New Jersey Medical School (CMDNJ), Newark, New Jersey 07103

JOSEPH CRAFT, Department of Ophthalmology and Visual Science, Yale University School of Medicine, 333 Cedar Street, New Haven, Connecticut 06510

JOHN E. DOWLING, The Biological Laboratories, Harvard University, Cambridge, Massachusetts 02138

RONALD W. EVERSON, School of Optometry, Indiana University, Bloomington, Indiana 47401

T. P. FLOOD, Department of Ophthalmology, Visual Physiology Laboratory (Retina Service), Jules Stein Eye Institute, UCLA School of Medicine, Los Angeles, California 90024

WARREN L. HERRON, JR., Department of Ophthalmology, University of Florida, Gainesville, Florida 32601

RUFUS HOWARD, Department of Ophthalmology and Visual Science, Yale University School of Medicine, 333 Cedar Street, New Haven, Connecticut 06510

LEE JAMPOL, Department of Ophthalmology and Visual Science, Yale University School of Medicine, 333 Cedar Street, New Haven, Connecticut 06510

ALBERT M. JONAS, Section of Comparative Medicine, Yale University School of Medicine, New Haven, Connecticut 06510

MOSHE LAHAV, Department of Ophthalmology and Visual Science, Yale University School of Medicine, 333 Cedar Street, New Haven, Connecticut 06510

YIN-LOK LAI, Section of Comparative Medicine, Yale University School of Medicine, New Haven, Connecticut 06510

MAURICE B. LANDERS, III, Duke University Eye Center, Durham, North Carolina 27710

ALAN M. LATIES, Department of Ophthalmology, Scheie Eye Institute, University of Pennsylvania Medical School, Philadelphia, Pennsylvania 19174

MATTHEW M. LAVAIL, Department of Neuropathology, Harvard Medical School, Department of Neuroscience, Children's Hospital Medical School, Boston, Massachusetts 02115

MICHAEL MARKOPOULOS, Department of Ophthalmology, New Jersey Medical School (CMDNJ), Newark, New Jersey 07103

EDWARD B. MCLEAN, Department of Ophthalmology, University of Washington, Seattle, Washington

RICHARD J. MULLEN, Department of Neuropathology, Harvard Medical School, Department of Neuroscience, Children's Hospital Medical School, Boston, Massachusetts 02115

WERNER K. NOELL, Neurosensory Laboratory, University of Buffalo, Buffalo, New York

JEROME T. PEARLMAN, Department of Ophthalmology, Visual Physiology Laboratory (Retina Service), Jules Stein Eye Institute, UCLA School of Medicine, Los Angeles, California 90024

J. SAXTON, Department of Medicine, UCLA School of Medicine, Los Angeles, California 90024

INGEBORG SCHMIDT, School of Optometry, Indiana University, Bloomington, Indiana 47401

S. R. SEIFF, Department of Ophthalmology, Visual Physiology Laboratory (Retina Service), Jules Stein Eye Institute, UCLA School of Medicine, Los Angeles, California 90024

DAVID H. SLINEY, Laser Microwave Division, U.S. Army Environmental Hygiene Agency, Aberdeen Proving Ground, Maryland 21010

GEORGE STEPHENS, Department of Ophthalmology, New Jersey Medical School (CMDNJ), Newark, New Jersey 07103

WILLIAM TENHOVE, Department of Medicine, New Jersey Medical School (CMDNJ), Newark, New Jersey 07103

M. O. M. TSO, Ophthalmic Pathology Division, Armed Forces Institute of Pathology, Washington, D.C. 20306

A. VAN HERLE, Department of Medicine, UCLA School of Medicine, Los Angeles, California 90024

JOSEPH A. C. WADSWORTH, Duke University Eye Center, Durham, North Carolina 27710

WILLIAM B. WATERS, North Carolina Division of Services for the Blind, PO Box 2658, Raleigh, North Carolina 27602

GEORGE W. WEINSTEIN, Division of Ophthalmology, University of Texas
    Health Science Center at San Antonio, San Antonio, Texas 78229

MYRON L. WOLBARSHT, Duke University Eye Center, Durham, North Caro-
    lina 27710

MITCHEL L. WOLF, The Jewish Hospital of St. Louis, Department of
    Ophthalmology, Washington University School of Medicine, 660
    South Euclid Avenue, St. Louis, Missouri 63110

RICHARD W. YOUNG, Department of Anatomy and Jules Stein Eye Insti-
    tute, UCLA School of Medicine, Los Angeles, California 90024

SECTION I

RETINITIS PIGMENTOSA: NATURAL HISTORY AND DIAGNOSIS

INTRODUCTION

Alan M. Laties

Department of Ophthalmology
Scheie Eye Institute
University of Pennsylvania Medical School
Philadelphia, Pennsylvania 19174

In starting this part of the program, I would like first of all to thank Drs. Wadsworth, Landers, and Wolbarsht for their very kind hospitality which all of us have enjoyed. It has been a wonderful experience to be here and see the manner in which this meeting has been run.

I also want to take a minute to make a few remarks on some efforts that are under way in trying to get some clinico-pathological material. Now, I am using clinico-pathological material in this case in a very broad sense. As you know, one of the great difficulties that all of us have is that we, at the moment, know more about the hereditary retinal degeneration of the RCS rat than we know about that of man. That is unfortunate. We want to know more about man. There are similarities between what happens in a particular animal and what occurs in man, but there is a real question as to how far these similarities go. The question is one of identity--are they identical? The question extends not only to this animal model but to all the others that are known. There are several people in this room who have worked in this area and one of the projects that is going on has been supported by the Retinitis Pigmentosa Foundation. The R. P. Foundation is currently trying to set up a donor eye program. In this program an attempt is being made to get first class histology at the EM level on eyes from patients with RP. The feasibility program is going on at the Berman-Gund Laboratory in Boston. I should tell you that Mr. Berman, the president of the R. P. Foundation is in the audience today. This study is being done

1

as an effort on the part of four or five individuals within the
laboratory. Each is willing to go out at all hours of the night to
do the taking of the eyes and to see to their preservation.

The R. P. Foundation would welcome any suggestions on how
this effort can be expanded. One idea that we have had is to get
together kits. We actually do have a kit, but it is very difficult
to accomplish the logistics. It is not an easy thing to get going.
Many of you know that there has been an effort of this type for ocular inflammations undertaken by the San Francisco group. They have
had some success at it.

The other RP effort being undertaken that may be of interest
to you is an attempt to get other animal models going. There is
now in Honey Brook, Pennsylvania, under the direction of Gustavo
Aguirre, an animal model program for dogs. We have several breeds
of dogs with hereditary retinal degenerations, the most successful
of which at the moment is Irish setters. From this effort, Irish
setters should be available shortly for researchers across the
country. They will be produced in very limited numbers, obviously,
and the cost will be substantial. But I think they will make a real
contribution. The sense of the effort is obvious--that every animal
model of hereditary retinal degeneration should be studied, and
studied in an intensive fashion.

THE NATURAL HISTORY OF RETINITIS PIGMENTOSA

George W. Weinstein

Division of Ophthalmology
University of Texas Health Science Center at San Antonio
San Antonio, Texas   78229

INTRODUCTION

Retinitis pigmentosa is a retinal degeneration characterized by night blindness, visual field constriction, and specific ophthalmoscopic and electrophysiological changes. Since its clinical course cannot be altered by any known form of treatment at the present time, it should be an easy task to elucidate the natural history of this disorder. However, because the progression of this condition is slow and often quite variable, even among affected family members, to do this properly would take decades of study (Sunga and Sloan, 1967).

This paper describes a different approach to the subject. A group of patients referred to a retinal function laboratory for evaluation has been studied with a series of diagnostic procedures. Most of the subjects were seen on only one occasion. For many, all of the indicated diagnostic procedures were performed, but for others, only a few were done. The results of these studies were correlated with age, sex, and subjective factors in an attempt to "reconstruct" the natural history of this condition.

SUBJECTS

The study population consisted of 139 subjects, 51% male and 49% female. Age range was from 2 to 82 years with a mean of 30 years (Table I). Further distribution of age of subjects by decade versus sex is given in Table II.

3

TABLE I

STUDY POPULATION

Number — 139

Sex   — 71 Male (51%)
            68 Female (49%)

Age   — 2-82 yrs. (mean = 30 yrs.)

TABLE II

AGE BY DECADES

1st	—	13 yrs.
2nd	—	30
3rd	—	32
4th	—	15
5th	—	23
≧6th	—	21
—	—	5

METHODS

The following diagnostic procedures were performed: (a) ophthalmologic history; (b) ophthalmoscopic examination; (c) electroretinography with constant amplitude and maximum intensity, single flash techniques; (d) electrooculography; (e) Goldmann-Weekers Dark Adaptometry; (f) Goldmann perimetry; and (g) fluorescein angiography.

The details of the techniques of each of these diagnostic procedures has been given in detail in previous publications (Forstot *et al.*, 1970; Lindquist *et al.*, 1970; Weinstein *et al.*, 1970, 1971; Reeser *et al.*, 1970; Hyvarinen *et al.*, 1969). Examples of data obtained by these various tests are given in Figs. 1-8.

RESULTS

The results of all of the diagnostic procedures were graded as shown in Table III.

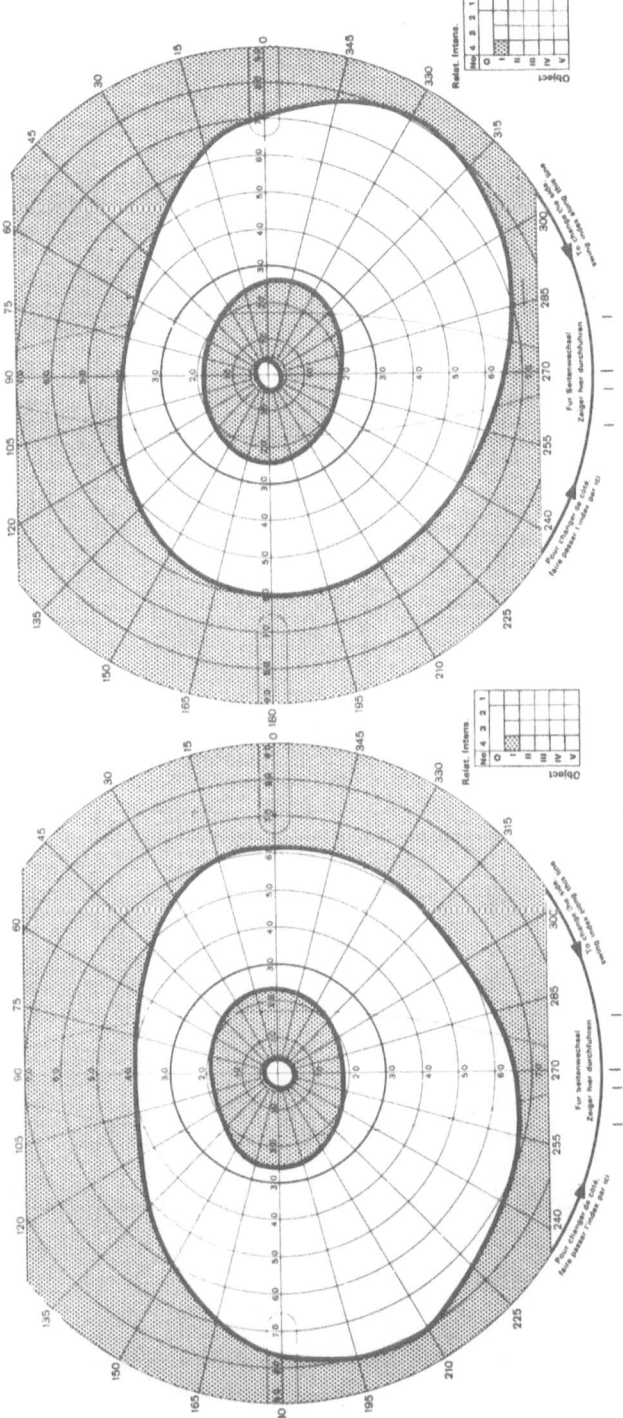

FIGURE 1. Visual fields performed with Goldmann perimeter on a 37 year old male with retinitis pigmentosa. Ring Scotoma is present.

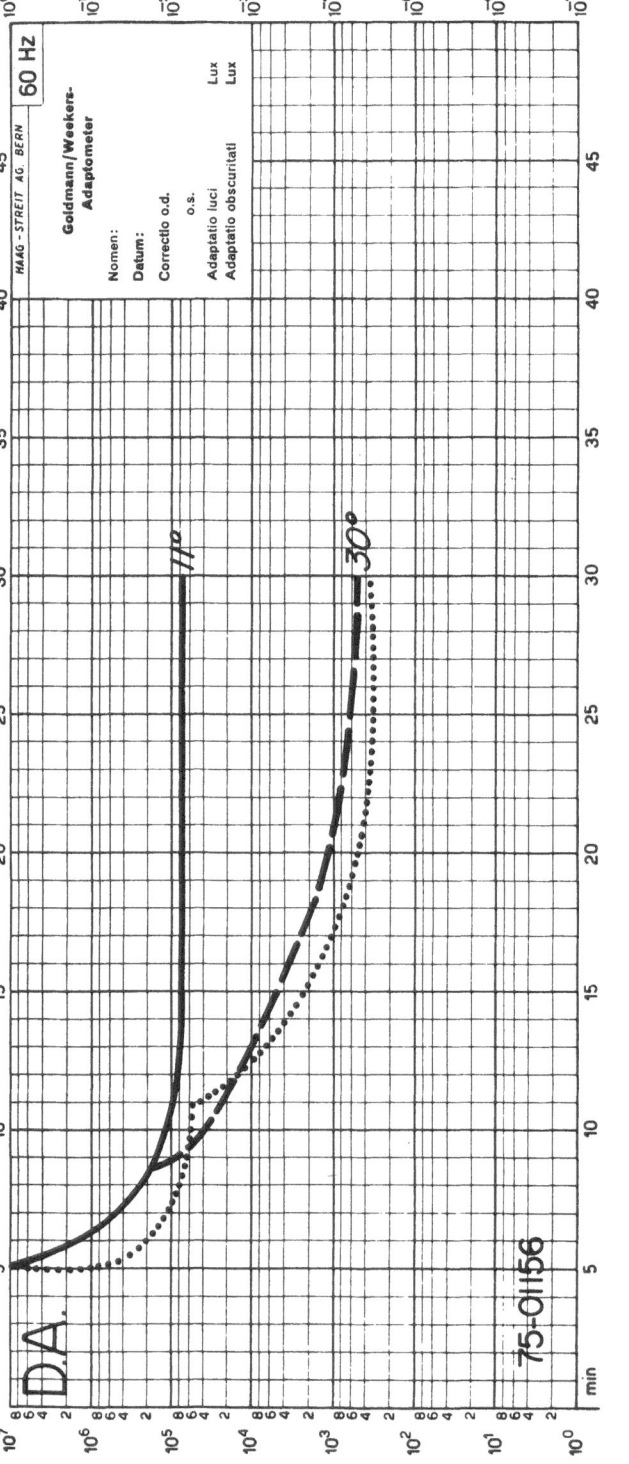

FIGURE 2. Dark adaptometry with Goldmann-Weeker's adaptometer, same subject as Fig. 1. Cone portion of curve shows mild elevation. Rod portion of curve is markedly elevated at 11° above fixation, but nearly normal 30° above fixation.

The grading of subjective symptoms is given in Table IV. The results are given in Table V. It is interesting to note that night blindness is not always appreciated by the subject, since many have been night blind since early childhood. Also, loss of peripheral visual field often goes unnoticed, since this occurs insidiously. The same may be true of color vision abnormalities. However, decreased visual acuity, which may occur early, is usually noted as soon as it occurs. Finally, patients often note photopsia (that is, flashes of light, as well as floaters in their visual surround). Note that the mean "severity" of the subjective symptoms is 2.5; that is between mild and moderate.

The grading method for dark adaptometry is shown in Table VI. The results of the subject study with dark adaptometry in our series is given in Table VII. Note that there were 18 individuals in this study who had normal dark adaptation studies. Of those who had dark adaptometry, the mean severity was 2.3, again between mild and moderate severity.

The grading of visual field studies is given in Table VIII. The characteristic ring scotoma has been designated as Grade 2 defect. Ten individuals had normal results, 20 had marked constriction (Table IX), and the mean was 2.5.

Table X shows the grading for the electroretinographic studies. Table XI gives the results of the ERG studies. Note that the non-recordable ERG, which is designated as Grade 4, includes 63 individuals. However, 30 subjects had normal ERG's and 33 had mild or moderately affected ERG's. Again, the mean severity falls between mild and moderate for this group.

TABLE III

Code for all parameters

0 Normal
1 Minimal or equivocal changes
2 Mild but definite changes
3 Moderate changes
4 Advanced changes
– Test not performed

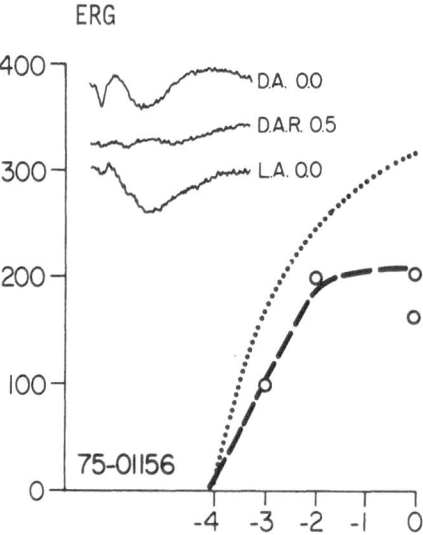

FIGURE 3. Electroretinography, same subject as Figs. 1 and 2.
Dark adapted responses to white and red light without and with
attenuating 0.5 log unit filter, respectively. Light adapted
responses are also shown, all in upper left portion of figure.
Intensity response curve is shown in lower right of figure,
with normal curve indicated with dotted line. Subject's subnormal curve is shown in dashed line. This patient's fundus
examination showed a moderate amount of bone spicule pigment
clumping in the mid-periphery.

        In an earlier study (Weinstein *et al.*, 1976), we compared the
relative sensitivity of electroretinography and dark adaptometry
performed with the Goldmann-Weekers instrument and with the Tubingen perimeter of Harms and Aulhorn. In that study, we found all
of these methods had approximately equal sensitivity for the detection of retinitis pigmentosa (Table XII).

        In Table XIII, the results are given for the 51 subjects who
had electrooculography studies. Most had either normal or markedly
affected EOG's, and the mean falls again between mild and moderately affected groups.

        The grading system for ophthalmoscopic changes is given in
Table XIV. One notes not only pigment clumping, but also areas of
depigmentation of the retinal pigment epithelium. Initially, the
optic disc is normal, but later in the disease, it assumes the
characteristic waxy pallor. Also, late in the disease, retinal

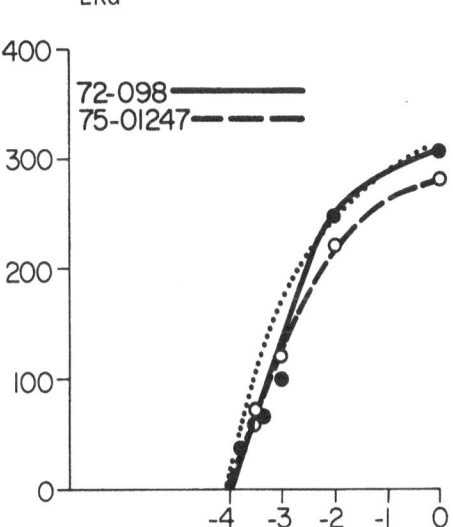

FIGURE 4. Intensity response curves of ERG b—wave amplitudes from 35 year old female with early retinitis pigmentosa. The solid curve is obtained from study performed three years prior to the dashed curve below it. The dotted line shows the normal ERG intensity response curve. This subject has dominantly inherited retinitis pigmentosa.

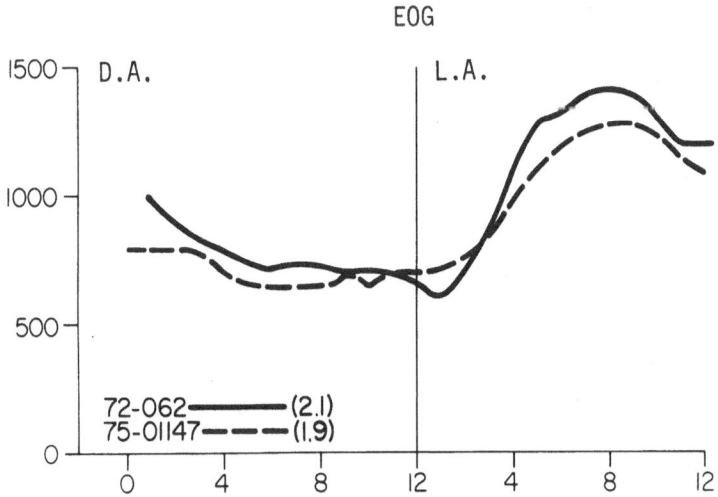

FIGURE 5. EOG recordings from same subject as in Fig. 4. Solid curve obtained from study performed in 1972, dashed curve obtained from study performed in 1975. EOG ratio has decreased from 2.1 to 1.9.

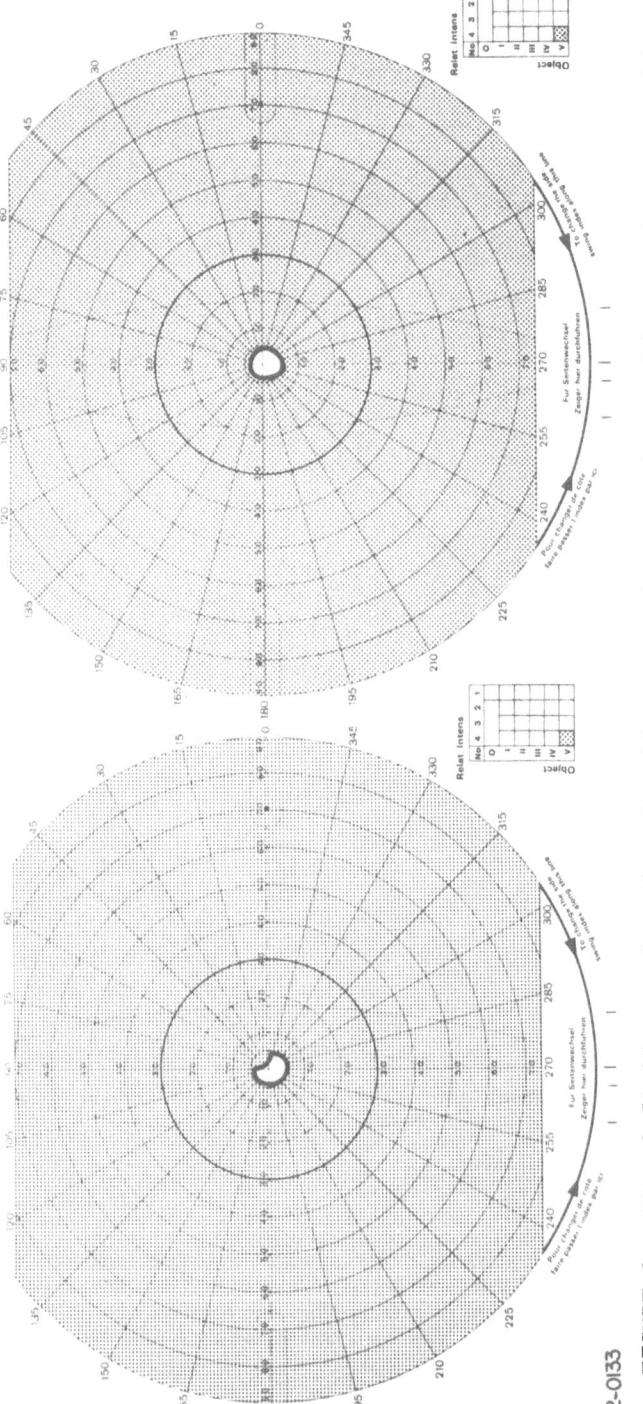

72-0133

FIGURE 6. Visual fields performed with Goldmann perimeter, from a 26 year old male subject with Laurence-Moon-Biedl syndrome and advanced retinitis pigmentosa. Only small central visual fields remain.

vessels, particularly the arterioles, become attenuated. The macula ordinarily is normal early in the disease, but atrophic changes may develop later.   Circulatory changes in the choroid are usually not visible ophthalmoscopically, and require fluorescein angiographic studies.   Table XV gives the results of our subjects with regard to ophthalmoscopic changes.   Note that 20 individuals had normal fundi and only 11 had markedly abnormal fundi. The mean severity here is 2.2.

ERG

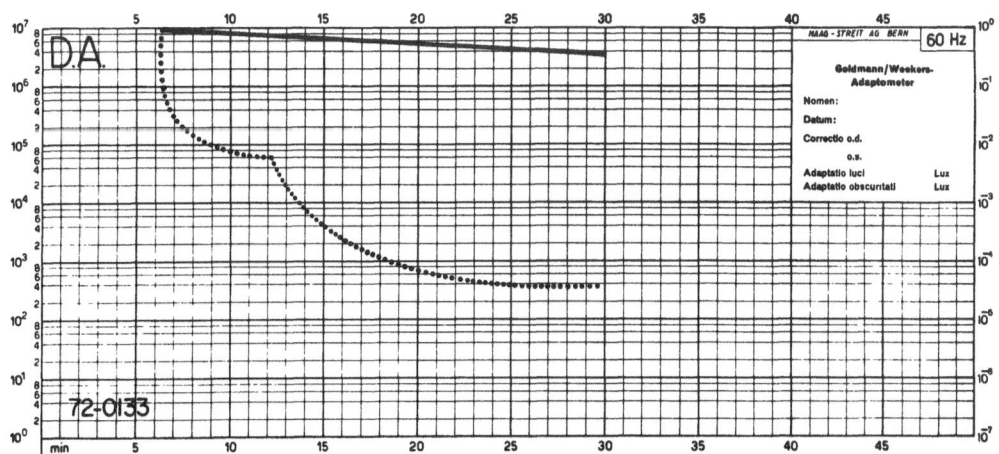

FIGURE 7.   Same subject as in Fig. 6.   ERG tracing above indicates that the response is non-recordable. Dark adaptometry below shows markedly elevated curve, solid line, above normal biphasic curve shown with dotted line below.

Relatively few patients in this study underwent fluorescein angiography. However, in earlier studies we have described some of the abnormalities which were noted again, and the grading of these changes is repeated in Table XVI. In addition to the pigmentary changes which are easily visible when highlighted with fluorescein, obvious circulatory changes can be noted, sometimes in very early cases. Areas of non-filling of the choriocapillaris are seen in some subjects, as well as areas in which the fluorescein dye persists for abnormally long periods of time. The results of the few subjects that we studied are given in Table XVII. It is important to note that these changes have often been noted even in subjects with early disease. As a result, it might be premature to discard the old concept that choroidal ischemia may be part of the pathogenetic mechanism, at least in some cases of retinitis pigmentosa.

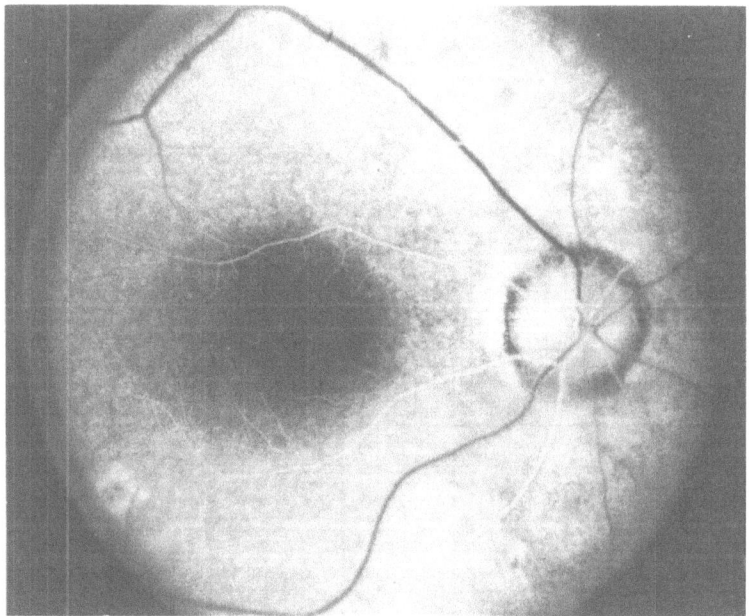

(FIGURE 8a)

FIGURE 8. Fluorescein angiography in a patient with moderately advanced retinitis pigmentosa. Early, late venous, and recirculation phases shown in a, b, and c, respectively. Note heavy accumulation of dye, persisting abnormally in latest phase.

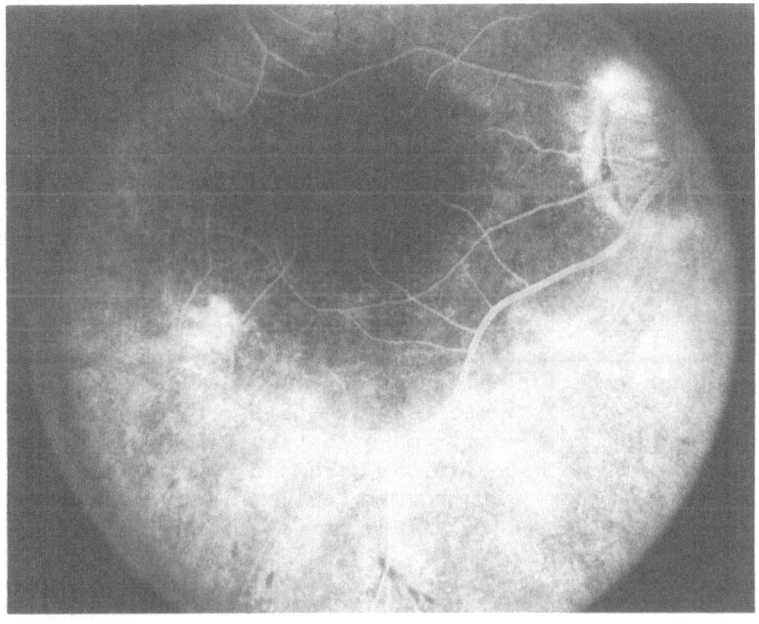

(FIGURE 8b)

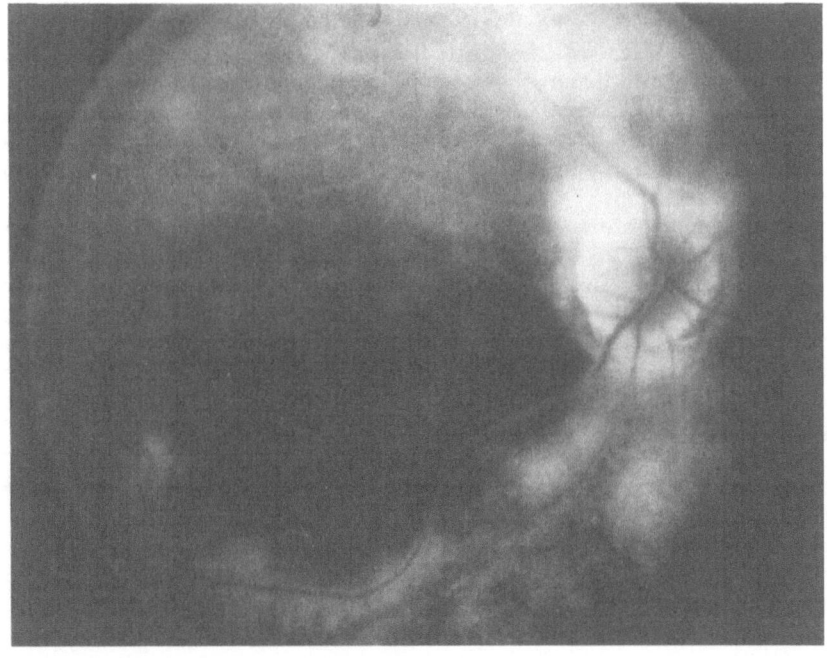

(FIGURE 8c)

Table XVIII gives the mean severity of each of the diagnostic studies in comparison to the subjects grouped by age and decades. It should be noted that through the first five decades of life, there is an even fixed distribution of subjects within each age group. Even more important, it is interesting that the mean severity in most of the groups remains much the same as one proceeds through the subjects by age. This either suggests that there is no progression in severity or that subjects have been referred at a fairly constant level of disease severity, probably the latter. Therefore, the data arranged in this way probably underlines the futility of attempting to define the natural history of retinitis pigmentosa in the way in which it has been attempted.

In another statistical approach using the Pearson product moment correlation (Sokal and Rohlf, 1969), we compared the severity of the subjective symptoms with those of the other tests. Although there was no correlation with age or with sex, there are positive correlations with regard to the ophthalmoscopic appearance, visual fields, dark adaptometry, electroretinography and electrooculography (Table XIX). That is, in this study, we could characterize the severity of the individual's disease just as well by eliciting the history carefully as we could by performing these other tests. None of the other diagnostic procedures were associated with as many positive correlations.

As a result of these studies, we have attempted to group our subjects into various stages of retinitis pigmentosa. Stage 0 would be considered the absence of disease; Stage 1, a mild disease; Stage 2, a moderate disease; and Stage 3, a severe disease. Accordingly, Table XX indicates that 9 individuals were normal in this series, 51 had severe disease, 12 had mild disease, and 67 had moderate disease. This staging was done on the basis of subjective symptoms alone. In testing the accuracy of staging the patients in this way, we also staged them according to three tests equally weighted--visual fields, dark adaptometry, and electroretinography--as well as to all seven tests equally weighted. Table XXI indicates that in 62 subjects, all three methods of staging agreed and that in 132 of the 139 cases, two of the three agreed. Table XXII summarizes the findings in the various stages of retinitis pigmentosa.

One should not leave the subject of retinitis pigmentosa without mentioning the fact that there are many factors mixed in, such as hereditary patterns of transmission, associated systemic and neurological conditions, as well as ocular abnormalities such as cataract, glaucoma and myopia.

TABLE IV

History

    0 No symptoms, no family history
    1 No symptoms, family history
    2 Night blind, normal photopic vision
    3 Night blind, affected photopic vision
    4 Poor or no vision

TABLE V

HISTORY – SEVERITY

0	–	0
1	–	15
2	–	23
3	–	70
4	–	4
–	–	26

← Mean = 2.5

TABLE VI

Dark-adapted studies

    0 Normal
    1 Isolated rod defect
    2 Widespread rod defects, mild
    3 Widespread rod defects, marked; normal cones
    4 Abnormal rods and cones

TABLE VII

DARK ADAPTOMETRY — SEVERITY

0	—	18
1	—	1
2	—	20
3	—	17
4	—	22
—	—	61

← Mean = 2.3

TABLE VIII

Light-adapted visual fields

0 Normal
1 Scattered relative scotomas
2 Ring scotoma
3 Generalized constriction, moderate
4 Generalized constriction, marked

TABLE IX

VISUAL FIELDS — SEVERITY

0	—	10
1	—	3
2	—	21
3	—	30
4	—	20
—	—	55

← Mean = 2.5

CONCLUSIONS

1. The pathogenesis of retinitis pigmentosa is still controversial.

2. The accurate recounting of the natural history of this disorder is difficult or impossible to do by single examinations of even large numbers of subjects, even when many different diagnostic procedures are performed. Only long term studies covering several decades are likely to accomplish this.

3. The severity of disease in given patients may be characterized easily, in this study with fair accuracy by the use of subjective symptoms alone, and with even greater accuracy when the results of other studies such as electroretinography, visual fields, and dark adaptometry are included. The ophthalmoscopic examination alone may be quite unreliable for the determination of severity of disease.

4. Retinitis pigmentosa is most likely a fundus response to any of a large number of initiating events rather than a single clinical entity. As such, it is unlikely that it would ever be curable, although it is conceivable that removal of the primary factors may result in its arrest or even reversal.

ACKNOWLEDGEMENTS

The author gratefully acknowledges the assistance of the following individuals: Andrew Biskin, for computer programming and statistical analysis; Gail Brogdon, for clerical support, Robert R. Hobson, for technical assistance; Cathy McKee, for manuscript preparation. The author is truly appreciative to each of the above for their help.

TABLE X

ERG

0 Normal
1 Subnormal threshold only
2 Subnormal scotopic, normal photopic responses
3 Subnormal scotopic and photopic responses
4 Non-recordable

TABLE XI

ERG – SEVERITY

0	–	30
1	–	4
2	–	15
3	–	18
4	–	63
–	–	9

← Mean = 2.6

TABLE XII

COMBINED STUDY

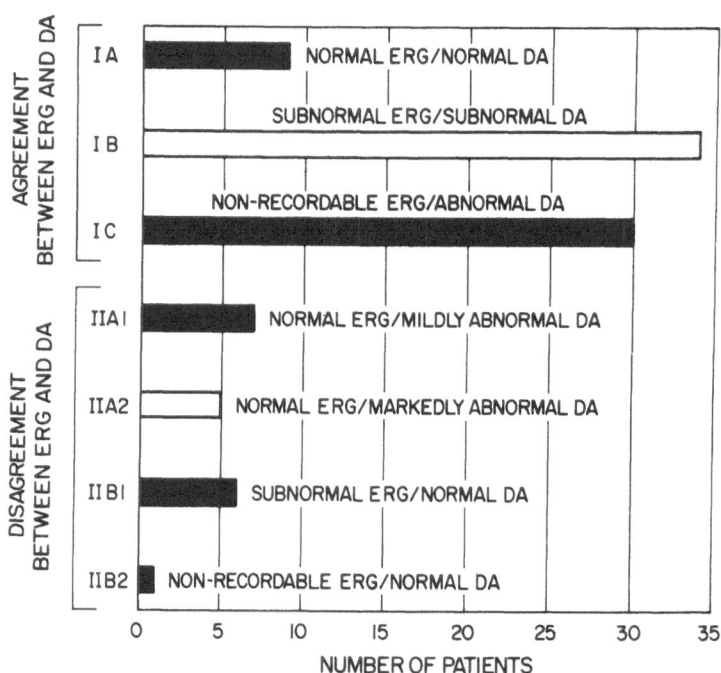

TABLE XIII

EOG – SEVERITY

0	–	18
1	–	0
2	–	3
3	–	8	← Mean = 2.3
4	–	22
–	–	88

TABLE XIV

Fundi

0 Normal
1 Rare pigmentary (or other) lesion
2 Obvious pigmentary changes, normal arterioles
3 Mild or marked pigmentary changes, with constricted arterioles
4 Advanced changes with optic atrophy

TABLE XV

FUNDI – SEVERITY

0	–	20
1	–	6
2	–	22
3	–	41	← Mean = 2.2
4	–	11
–	–	39

TABLE XVI

Fluorescein angiography

0   Normal
1   Minimal pigmentary or circulatory changes
2   Definite abnormalities of choriocapillaris
3   Choroidal atrophy in some areas
4   Marked changes in choroidal circulation

TABLE XVII

FLUORESCEIN ANGIOGRAPHY – SEVERITY

$$
\begin{array}{ccc}
0 & - & 3 \\
1 & - & 4 \\
2 & - & 4 \\
3 & - & 1 \\
4 & - & 5 \\
- & - & 122 \\
\end{array}
$$

← Mean = 2.1

TABLE XVIII

CORRELATIONS WITH AGE BY DECADE

		Age	Sex	Hist.	Fundi	VF	DA	ERG	EOG
Decade	1	5.7	1.2	2.6	2.1	3.0	2.4	2.8	–
	2	14.0	1.4	2.5	1.8	2.2	2.4	2.2	1.6
	3	24.0	1.6	2.3	2.1	2.6	1.7	2.9	2.6
	4	34.6	1.5	2.8	2.4	2.7	2.4	2.4	1.8
	5	44.1	1.4	2.7	2.6	2.5	2.8	2.7	2.2
	≥ 6	62	1.7	2.6	2.2	2.8	2.7	2.6	3.2

TABLE XIX

CORRELATIONS WITH HISTORY

		Age	Sex	Fundi	VF	DA	ERG	EOG
History	1	23	1.5	.3	.2	0.0	.4	0.0
by	2	32	1.4	1.7	2.3	1.6	3.0	2.3
grade	3	30	1.6	2.6	2.9	3.1	2.9	3.0
	4	28	1.5	3.3	3.0	3.0	4.0	4.0
	All	30	1.5	2.2	2.6	2.3	2.6	2.3
Correlation →		−0.02	−0.02	.4	.4	.7	.4	.4

TABLE XX

STAGING PATIENTS IN SERIES
(Correlated to History)

Stage	0 (no disease)	9
	1 (mild)	12
	2 (moderate)	67
	3 (severe)	51

TABLE XXI

STAGING PATIENTS IN SERIES

History vs. VF + DA + ERG
and
History vs. All 7 tests

	Agree all 3, by quintiles:	62
plus	Agree 2/3, by quintiles:	70
	No 2 agree:	7

TABLE XXII

Stage 0: early abnormalities of scotopic vision and/or suggestive angiographic findings.

Stage 1: widespread abnormalities of scotopic vision with normal or slightly abnormal photopic vision.

Stage 2: widespread abnormalities of photopic vision with normal or slightly abnormal ophthalmoscopic findings.

Stage 3: advanced psychophysical, electrophysiological and ophthalmoscopic findings.

0: Normal, ±: minimally or equivocally affected, +: mildly affected, ++: definitely affected, +++: severely affected.

REFERENCES

Forstot, L., Weinstein, G., and Feiock, K. (1970) Studies with the Tubingen perimeter of Harms and Aulhorn. *Ann. Ophthal.* 2:843-854.

Hyvarinen, L., Maumenee, A. E., George, T., and Weinstein, G. W. (1969) Fluorescein angiography of the choriocapillaris. *Amer. J. Ophthal.* 67:653-666.

Lindquist, C., Weinstein, G. W., and Feiock, K. (1970) Absolute profile fields in normal subjects and in early cases of retinitis pigmentosa. *EENT Monthly* 49:45-54.

Reeser, F., Weinstein, G. W., and Feiock, K. (1970) The normal and supernormal electrooculogram. *Amer. J. Ophthal.* 70:505-514.

Sokal, R. R., and Rohlf, F. J. (1969) "Biometry," W. H. Freeman, San Francisco, p. 498.

Sunga, R. N., and Sloan, L. L. (1967) Pigmentary degeneration of the retina: Early diagnosis and natural history. *Invest. Ophthal.* 6:309-325.

Weinstein, G. W., Weinberg, R., and Hobson, R. (1970) Constant amplitude electroretinography as a test of retinal sensitivity in normal and abnormal subjects. *Amer. J. Ophthal.* 69:836-849.

Weinstein, G. W., Maumenee, A. E., and Hyvarinen, L. (1971) On the pathogenesis of retinitis pigmentosa. *Ophthalmologica* 162: 82-97.

Weinstein, G. W., Lowell, G. G., and Hobson, R. R. (1976) A comparison of electroretinographic and dark adaptation studies in retinitis pigmentosa. *Documenta Ophthalmologica* (in press).

DISCUSSION OF THE PAPER

DR. BRADBURY: Did you find any association with keratoconus? I know there have been several reports saying that there is an association.

DR. WEINSTEIN: I think we had two patients with keratoconus in our series and there have been individual instances, but those are just kind of anecdotal events.

DR. SCHMIDT: I feel uneasy when doing dark adaptation tests because I believe that light is damaging, and therefore I don't like to do dark adaptation tests on retinitis pigmentosa patients.

DR. WEINSTEIN: Well, we also examine these patients with the indirect ophthalmoscope and we do fluorescein angiography, so if light is damaging we are damaging a great number of patients. I hope it is not.

DR. SIEGEL: Could a good substitute for dark adaptation simply be dark adapting the patient previously and then doing threshold measurements just to get the final absolute thresholds? That is really better than dark adaptation without any light adaptation at all.

DR. SCHMIDT: I agree.

DR. WEINSTEIN: Well, perhaps all you have to do is take a careful history, remember.

DR. DOWLING: In the dark!

ELECTRORETINOGRAPHY AND THE DIAGNOSIS OF RETINITIS PIGMENTOSA

Jerome T. Pearlman

Department of Ophthalmology, Visual Physiology Laboratory
(Retina Service), Jules Stein Eye Institute
UCLA School of Medicine
Los Angeles, California 90024

The electroretinogram (ERG) is the graphic representation of an electrical mass response of the retina to light stimulation of brief duration. As such, the ERG is an objective measurement of retinal function. Like the electrocardiogram, the ERG is a complex wave form, consisting of a number of component potentials. Over the years, numerous efforts have been made to analyze the electro-retinographic response, and to break down the complex wave form into the various component parts. One classic analysis of the ERG was set forth by Granit (1933), who defined three component processes (P_1, P_{11}, and P_{111}), named in the order in which they disappeared under ether anesthesia. Roughly speaking, the P_1 process was equivalent to the c-wave, the P_{11} equivalent to the b-wave, and the P_{111} equivalent to the a-wave. These designations are now considered to be primarily of historic interest. Alphabetical letters designating various portions of the complex wave form (i.e., a-, b-, c-, and d-waves) owe their origin to Einthoven and Jolly (1908).

Despite the fact that the electroretinogram had been known as a biologic entity since 1865, Karpe, in 1945, was the first to report an "extinguished" ERG in primary pigmentary degeneration of the retina. With respect to retinitis pigmentosa in its various forms, the common absence of the ERG response is now considered to be as important a diagnostic criterion as pigmentary changes within the retina, arteriolar attenuation, and waxy pallor of the optic disc. Thus, the ERG becomes an important tool in the differentiation of primary pigmentary retinal degeneration from other similar appearing, but secondary syndromes, where the ERG may be normal, subnormal, but not totally absent.

As a diagnostic procedure, the ERG can be performed in young individuals, albeit under sedation or general anesthesia; whereas visual field testing or dark adaptometry may not be possible owing to lack of cooperation. The differential use of the electroretinogram was further emphasized by Karpe (1945) and Francois (1951), who proposed that the ERG would allow one to predict which asymptomatic members of affected families would ultimately suffer from primary pigmentary degeneration. Berson *et al.* (1969) and others have drawn attention, again, to the temporal aspects of the electroretinogram, as exemplified by the implicit time or culmination time, and the prognostic value of this parameter.

Amplitude changes in the electroretinogram may be highly variable, and are not necessarily due to pathologic alterations of retinal function. Therefore, conclusions regarding the abnormality of the electroretinographic response, based purely on diminished response amplitudes, are fraught with possibilities for error, unless certain qualifications are made. Clearly, averaged amplitudes are more reliable in a quantitative sense than are the amplitude measurements of single flash responses; and values derived from slope functions are, again, more stable and reliable than individual flash amplitudes.

It has been recognized for some years that the time related aspects of the ERG response are more stable, and hence, better indicators of normalcy. Changes in latency and culmination times are known to be more closely related to pathologic alterations of the retina than changes in wave heights. Similarly, threshold determinations of ERG response, particularly in the dark-adapted state, are more significant than amplitude changes, since the former are more closely related to the rhodopsin content of rod outer segments.

Summation of ERG responses employing the biologic computer of average transients (C.A.T.) is an important advance in clinical testing. While not absolutely essential for routine electroretinography, computer averaging techniques are almost mandatory for the visual evoked response (VER).

Use of the term "extinguished" ERG is to be avoided. "Non-recordability" is preferred, since the latter implies an artifact of our recording technique, and not the direct consequence of the disease process. ERG responses that are "non-recordable" by single flash techniques are almost invariably "recordable" when summation and averaging are used.

While electroretinographic changes are usually extreme in primary retinitis pigmentosa, they are not invariably so. Some degree of response impairment is almost universally present: typically, the scotopic b-wave is severely diminished or non-recordable.

There are many reports of "non-extinguished" potentials, particularly with preservation of the a-wave, but much depends on the recording techniques, the duration of the disease, and even the mode of genetic transmission. Persons having the autosomal dominant form of the disease are said to have a later onset of their symptoms and milder, less rapidly progressive functional loss. There is some evidence now, however, that the autosomal dominant form of retinitis pigmentosa is more pleomorphic than heretofore believed.

The electroretinogram, as a diagnostic procedure, is probably not necessary in the routine case of typical retinitis pigmentosa, since the mere presence of pigmentary change indicates an advanced state of the disorder. In terms of following a patient with established retinitis pigmentosa, the ERG is perhaps the least valuable of the routine function tests. Once the ERG is gone, it is gone.

Progression of the disease is better documented with Goldmann fields and dark adaptometry. As stated earlier, the ERG may be helpful in identifying early functional changes in persons having a family history of retinitis pigmentosa, but showing few, if any, of the clinical features of the disease itself.

The electroretinogram cannot really be used to classify patients according to the degree of functional disability. Arden and Fojas (1962) were unable to find any correlation between the visual field, visual acuity and the possibility of obtaining an ERG. It was their conclusion that the electrooculogram (EOG) was a better diagnostic tool with respect to retinitis pigmentosa than the ERG.

From the work of Francois and De Rouck (1962), we know the following about the ERG and the changes it undergoes in various pathologic circumstances, particularly in retinitis pigmentosa: (1) The ERG response is not always absent. (2) Early, there may be a "subnormal" or impaired response, short of total non-recordability. (3) The presence of a normal ERG response, especially in infants, does not permit the exclusion of the diagnosis of retinitis pigmentosa, nor does it imply that the eyes are normal.

The ERG, together with other functional tests, including the EOG, is still essential in establishing the diagnosis in non-pigmented retinitis pigmentosa, or in atypical cases.

In summary, the ERG remains an important tool in the diagnosis of primary pigmentary retinal degeneration, despite certain acknowledged limitations. It has a certain predictive value. In the last analysis, the electroretinogram is but one of a variety of diagnostic techniques we have at our disposal. The ERG has to be used in conjunction with other function tests, including visual acuity, fields, dark adaptation, and color vision testing, to clarify and classify a variety of retinal disorders.

ACKNOWLEDGEMENTS

This study was supported by NIH grant EY 00331, from the National Eye Institute (Bethesda, Maryland), and from the private contributions of the Sklar and Phillips families (Shreveport, Louisiana).

REFERENCES

Arden, G. B., and Fojas, M. R. (1962) Electrophysiological abnormalities in pigmentary degenerations of the retina. Assessment of values and basis. *Arch. Ophthal.* 68(3):369-389.

Berson, E. L., Gouras, P., and Hoff, M. (1969) Temporal aspects of the electroretinogram. *Arch. Ophthal.* 81(2):207-214.

Einthoven, W., and Jolly, W. (1908) The form and magnitude of the electrical responses of the eye to stimulation by light at various intensities. *Quart. J. Exp. Physiol.* 1:373.

Francois, J. (1951) Premiers essais d'electroretinographie clinique. *Bull. Soc. belg. Ophthal.* 99:457-470.

Francois, J., and De Rouck; A. (1962) The use of twin flashes in electroretinography. Characteristics of the electroretinogram in normal cases and in choriodoretinal heredodegenerations. *Amer. J. Ophthal.* 54(1):54-63.

Granit, R. (1933) The components of the retinal action potential and their relation to the discharge in the optic nerve. *J. Physiol. (Lond.)* 77:207-240.

Karpe, G. (1945) The basis of clinical electroretinography. *Acta Ophthal. (Kbh.)* Suppl. 23, 1-114.

DISCUSSION OF THE PAPER

DR. JOONDEPH: Have you found any correlation whatsoever between visual fields and ERG and EOG? In those institutions where the ERG is not available can the practitioner make a diagnosis with the use of a visual field and without using the ERG or EOG?

DR. PEARLMAN: I think the visual field is extremely helpful. I also think that a history of night blindness is very significant. If you get a history of night blindness with tubular fields or with constriction of the inner isopters, I think that is very important. The visual fields can be used to show a progression of the disease, but I don't find that they correlate terribly well with the ERG. Not in a precise way. I am really in love with the dark adaptation test, despite the fact that we may feel that it is a psychophysical test and subjective and can't be relied upon because of differences in people. With a cooperative subject it is an exquisite test of retinal function.

DR. RICKER: Is ERG equipment standardized throughout the country?

DR. PEARLMAN: No.

DR. RICKER: Why?

DR. PEARLMAN: First, there is a limited demand for such instrumentation. Second, each investigator seeks to acquire specialized information from the ERG. This means the recording methods will vary in accordance with the data desired.

DR. SANDBERG: Can you distinguish between stationary night blindness and RP with just dark adaptation?

DR. PEARLMAN: No.

DR. DOWLING: I think that the question before last is a very important one. Virtually everybody doing ERG's around the country does them differently--they use different equipment, different criteria to record, to stimulate the retina, what have you, and I think that until one brings some standardization into this whole field that it is going to be very difficult to compare studies between laboratories. I think this is a very important point and I think this is something we are going to have to do in the reasonably near future in order to make sense out of this whole business.

DR. PEARLMAN: True, but thus far no single means of recording the ERG is clearly superior to all others.

THE CLINICAL SIGNIFICANCE OF RETINITIS PIGMENTOSA WITHOUT PIGMENT:

A COMPUTER ASSISTED ANALYSIS

J. T. Pearlman, J. Saxton, T. P. Flood and S. R. Seiff

Department of Ophthalmology, Visual Physiology Laboratory
(Retina Service), Jules Stein Eye Institute
UCLA School of Medicine
Los Angeles, California 90024

INTRODUCTION

The purpose of this report is to reiterate and lend statistical validity to the concept that retinitis pigmentosa without
fundus pigment is not a rare or unusual form of the disease, but
quite likely the initial stage of typical retinitis pigmentosa
(Nettleship, 1908, 1914; Leber, 1871, 1877; Gebb, 1909).   As such,
the non-pigmented state is manifested by shorter duration of symptoms, less severe night blindness, and less impairment of the
electroretinographic b-wave.

MATERIALS AND METHODS

The subjects analyzed in this study are the first 68 consecutive patients to be entered into the Jules Stein Eye Institute
Retinitis Pigmentosa Registry for Southern California.   The Registry is an ongoing activity recording all patients bearing the
diagnosis of primary pigmentary retinal degeneration seen at the
Jules Stein Eye Institute since November, 1974.   The findings for
each patient are recorded on a special data sheet.   That information is, in turn, transferred to IBM punchcards for computer
processing.   Our method for data gathering has been previously
described (Peterson *et al*., 1970).

The data sheets began with patient identification and general
information.   Pertinent history was recorded noting, among other
things, the mode of genetic inheritance, the age of the patient at
the onset of night blindness, and any significant history relating

31

to drug ingestion or medication. The duration of the disease was defined, for our purposes, as the patient's present age minus the age at the onset of night blindness. As the data sheets were completed, the information was transferred to IBM punchcards. Statistical evaluation was performed, using an IBM 360/91 computer at the Health Sciences Computing Facility, University of California, Los Angeles.

Patients having typical retinitis pigmentosa are defined as those with a history of night blindness, elevated rod threshold by dark adaptation, bilaterally constricted visual fields, bilateral ERG b-wave abnormalities, typical bilateral mid-peripheral or peripheral retinal pigmentation of the bone corpuscular variety, and fluorescein angiographic evidence of retinal pigment epithelial disease.

Patients failing to show pigmentation within the retina, but who may have a family history of the disease, or the characteristic physiopathologic findings, are categorized as having retinitis pigmentosa without pigment. While there are, undoubtedly, several categories of retinitis pigmentosa without pigment (Berson, 1969, 1972), they are considered together for the purpose of this study. [Leber (1871), who was the first to describe retinitis pigmentosa with minimal or absent pigment, named that condition "retinitis pigmentosa sine pigmento." Undoubtedly, he was referring to those patients with far-advanced disease, showing attenuation of the retinal arterioles and waxy pallor of the optic nerve heads. Such patients, even after many years, failed to develop the pigmentary changes characteristic of the disease. Another category of retinitis pigmentosa patients, also without pigment, may have a long history of night blindness, rapid progression of visual difficulty, but no ophthalmoscopically evident fundus abnormalities.]

RESULTS

Fifteen of our 68 patients (22%) had the non-pigmented form of the disease. The various genetic modes of inheritance occurred with the following frequencies: 5.9% were autosomal dominant; 7.4% X-linked recessive; 13.2% autosomal recessive; and 73.5% sporadic. If the autosomal recessive group was combined with the sporadic, on the basis that the two most likely represent the same form of autosomal recessive inheritance, the frequency was 86.7%. Fifty-two percent were males, 48% females.

An F distribution test was used to determine whether there was a significant difference in the duration of symptoms in patients with the non-pigmented form of the disease, as opposed to patients having characteristic pigment deposition within the retina. The test showed a statistically significant difference between the mean duration of symptoms of these two populations, p<0.05. As the duration of night blindness increased, the percentage of patients with retinitis pigmentosa without pigment decreased. For patients with a history of night blindness of three years or less, 50% were of the non-pigmented variety. When the history of night vision difficulty was present for up to 15 years, the percentage of non-pigmented cases dropped to 16.5%. Overall, the incidence of retinitis pigmentosa without visible evidence of pigment was 22%.

Further analysis revealed that the electroretinograms of retinitis pigmentosa patients without pigment were significantly less impaired than those with pigment (chi square test, p<0.005). If one considered only right eyes, 50% of the non-pigmented group had abnormal but recordable ERG's, while only 8.9% of the patients with pigmentation had this type of ERG change. Fifty percent of the non-pigmented group had non-recordable ERG's, as opposed to 84% of those showing typical pigmentary change. The results were very much the same when only left eyes were considered.

Moreover, there was a statistically significant difference between the two groups of patients with respect to dark adaptation function. Those without pigment had less elevation of the final rod threshold than those with pigmentation; using the Fischer's exact test, p<0.05.

DISCUSSION

This study supports the impression of earlier investigators that retinitis pigmentosa begins without ophthalmoscopically observable pigment. The validity of the sample in this study is demonstrated by the agreement of our data with previously established values for the relative frequency of the various modes of inheritance and the slight predominance of males over females due to X-linked recessive transmission (Duke-Elder and Dobree, 1967).

The duration of symptoms for retinitis pigmentosa without pigment is significantly lower than for the pigmented stage of the disease. The incidence of retinitis pigmentosa without pigment is highest when the duration of symptoms is less than three years. The percentage of non-pigmented cases decreases as the duration of symptoms lengthens, but maintains an overall average of 22%.

If a non-pigmented form of retinitis pigmentosa can signify an early stage of the disease, one can understand why night vision impairment might be less severe, and why there might be less functional impairment of the ERG response. These findings, however, do not preclude the existence--in certain instances--of cases of retinitis pigmentosa without pigment that show marked loss of visual fields, rapid progression of the disease, and severe functional disturbance. We know that such cases exist (Goodman and Gunkel, 1958).

At any time between the onset of night blindness and 20 or more years following, the patient may begin to show pigment deposition within the retina. The exact time at which pigment appears, however, is highly variable. In RCS (Royal College of Surgeons) dystrophic rats having hereditary pigmentary retinal degeneration resembling retinitis pigmentosa, intraretinal pigment migration occurs late in the disease, after the ERG has become non-recordable and severe changes have occurred in the anatomic structure of the rod outer segments (Dowling and Sidman, 1962).

Clinicians should suspect retinitis pigmentosa, even in the absence of pigmentary changes, if there is a family history of the disease; or, if there is night blindness; ophthalmoscopic evidence of retinal arteriolar attenuation, with or without waxy pallor of the optic disc; and peripheral field constriction. Pigment deposition, in and of itself, is of secondary importance, apart from enabling the clinician to make a diagnosis without resorting to special tests of visual function.

SUMMARY

Sixty-eight consecutive patients with retinitis pigmentosa were studied to determine the frequency of the non-pigmented form of the disease. There was an overall incidence of 22%.

Fifty percent of all cases had no characteristic pigmentation, if the duration of night vision difficulty was three years or less.

The study lends statistical support to the concept that the non-pigmented form of retinitis pigmentosa is frequently an early stage of the disease and not an unusual or atypical variant. Patients without the pigmentary changes characteristic of the disorder also showed less functional impairment: the ERG b-wave was more apt to be recordable, although impaired; and the rod threshold, as determined by dark adaptation measurement, was less elevated.

The clinician should suspect retinitis pigmentosa, even in the absence of pigmentary changes, if there is a family history of the disorder, night blindness, peripheral field loss, and an impaired or non-recordable electroretinographic response.

ACKNOWLEDGEMENTS

We are grateful to the Health Sciences Computing Facility, UCLA, for computing assistance, supported by NIH special research sources grant RR-3; and to Mrs. Nola J. Allston and Mr. Robert Petrus for technical assistance. This study was supported by NIH grant EY 00331, from the National Eye Institute (Bethesda, Maryland), and from the private contributions of the Sklar and Phillips Families (Shreveport, Louisiana).

REFERENCES

Berson, E. L. (1969) Retinitis pigmentosa without pigment (Editorial). *Arch. Ophthal.* 81:453.

Berson, E. L. (1972) Electroretinographic testing as an aid in determining visual prognosis in families with hereditary retinal degenerations, in "Retina Congress" Chapter 3, p. 41, Appleton-Century-Crofts, New York.

Dowling, J. E., and Sidman, R. L. (1962) Inherited retinal dystrophy in the rat. *J. Cell. Biol.* 14:73.

Duke-Elder, S., and Dobree, J. H. (1967) "System of Ophthalmology, Vol. X, Diseases of the Retina," p. 577, C. V. Mosby, St. Louis.

Gebb, H. (1909) Zur Casuistik der Retinitis pigmentosa sine pigmento. *Arch. f. Augenheilkunde* 64:204.

Goodman, G., and Gunkel, R. D. (1958) Familial electroretinographic and adaptometric studies in retinitis pigmentosa. *Amer. J. Ophthal.* 46:142 (Sept., Part II).

Leber, T. (1871) Ueber anomale Formen der Retinitis pigmentosa. *Graefe's Arch. f. Ophthal.* 17(1):314.

Leber, T. (1877) in "Graefe-Saemisch Handbuch der gesamten Augenheilkunde" (ed. 1), Vol. 5, Engelmann, Leipzig.

Nettleship, E. (1908) On retinitis pigmentosa and allied diseases. *Roy. Lond. Ophthal. Hosp. Rep.* 17 (pt. 3):365.

Nettleship, E. (1914) A note on the progress of some cases of retinitis pigmentosa sine pigmento and retinitis punctata albescens. *Roy. Lond. Ophthal. Hosp. Rep.* 19 (pt. 2):123.

Peterson, N. D., Pearlman, J. R., Straatsma, B. R., and Bauschek, E. K. (1970) Diabetic retinopathy and computer processing. *Amer. J. Ophthal.* 70:548.

RETINITIS PIGMENTOSA AND A RETINAL VASCULOPATHY OF THE COATS TYPE

W. Banks Anderson, Jr., Joseph A. C. Wadsworth, and
Maurice B. Landers

Duke University Eye Center
Durham, North Carolina 27710

Primary pigmentary degenerations of the retina (the retinitis pigmentosa group of diseases) have been associated with many central nervous system afflictions. The association of retinitis pigmentosa with drusen of the optic disc and with posterior subcapsular cataracts is also well known. Not so well known, however, is the association between retinitis pigmentosa and a vasculopathy of the retina with the clinical appearance of Coats's disease.

We wish to describe a patient with exudative retinal vasculopathy and retinitis pigmentosa. Although we can discover only six other similar cases in the world's literature, we suspect that the association of these two diseases is more common than these few reports would indicate.

A 22-year-old farm worker was initially seen at the Duke University Eye Center complaining of difficulty with night vision for as long as he could remember. No other member of the family was so affected. He had been fitted with spectacles at age 5 and subsequently was seen by many different ophthalmologists. In his first examination at the Duke Eye Center, he was found to have a best corrected visual acuity of 20/200 in the right eye and 20/80 in the left, bilateral 10° visual fields, and the typical clinical picture of retinitis pigmentosa. There was waxy optic atrophy and bone spicule pigmentation bilaterally. An unusual and unexpected finding, however, was the presence of vascular telangiectasis and retinal and subretinal exudate in the periphery of both eyes (Fig. 1). Exudate was also present about the right optic disc with exudative detachment at the right macula typical of the picture seen in Coats's disease. There were anterior and posterior subcapsular cataracts and the vitreous seemed to have more strands and veils than in the usual patient of this age. The electroretinogram was extinguished and the electrooculogram was grossly depressed.

37

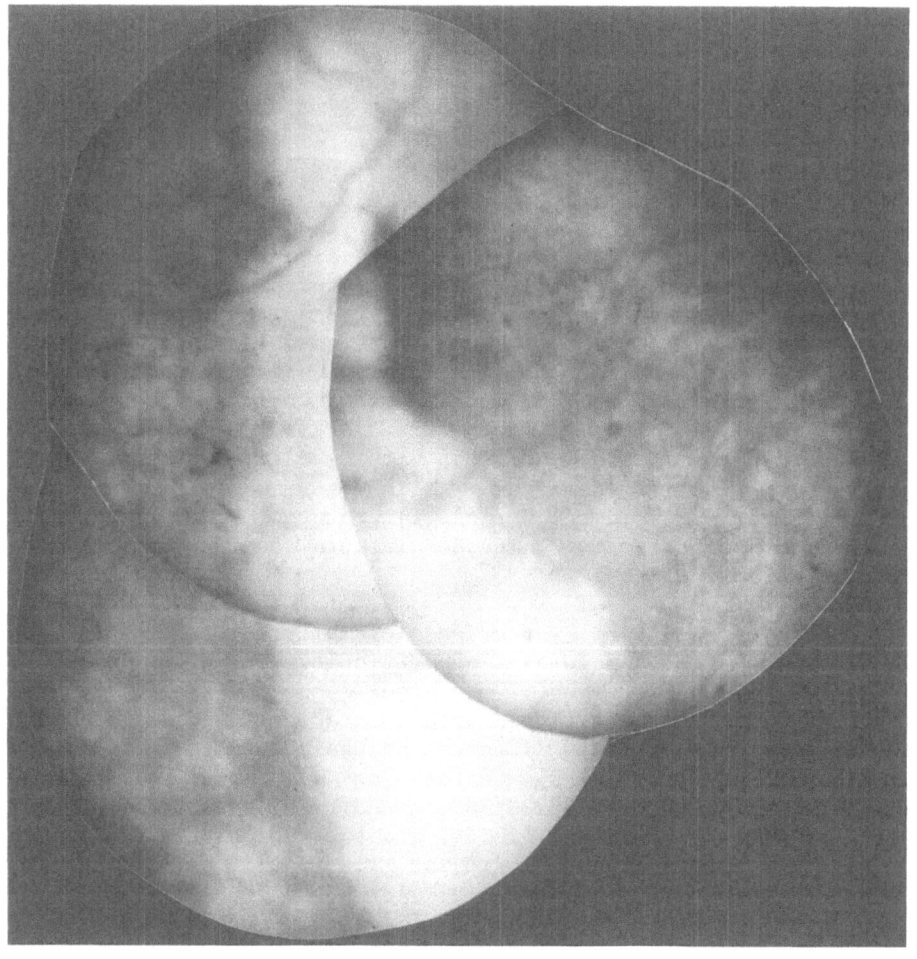

FIGURE 1. Periphery of right eye demonstrating bone spicule pig-
         mentation and retinal exudate.

Responses to the Farnsworth D-15 panel suggested tritanopia. Dark adaptation was grossly abnormal with no demonstrable final rod or cone threshold or transition time. Urine amino acid analysis and 17 hydroxy and 17 ketosteroid analysis revealed a normal adult pattern while serum cholesterol, triglycerides, and lipoproteins were also normal. Serologic tests for syphilis were negative, as were the hemogram, urinalysis, and glucose tolerance tests.

It was felt that the areas of peripheral vascular abnormality in the right eye might benefit from cryosurgical treatment and this was performed uneventfully. Six months following treatment, visual acuity had improved from 20/200 to 20/80 and the retina appeared flatter with less exudate. The untreated left eye remained unchanged.

In a review of the medical literature we have discovered six other similar cases (Zamorani, 1956; Morgan and Crawford, 1968; Schmidt and Faulborn, 1970; Egerer et al., 1974). The data from these reports and from our case are summarized in Table I. Although the retinal appearance in these cases is quite typical of what most ophthalmologists know as Coats's disease, Type II (Wise et al., 1971), there are several features of our case and of the reported cases which do not fit the usual clinical pattern in this disease.

Whereas Coats's disease is ordinarily seen three times more frequently in males than in females, in our collected series there is a preponderance of females. The usual Coats patient is affected in only one eye; however, in all but one of the patients with retinitis pigmentosa whose fundus could be seen, the condition was present bilaterally. Although Coats's disease is occasionally seen in adult life, most of the cases are diagnosed during childhood. In our series, the youngest patient was 16 years of age. These differences suggest that the etiology of the vasculopathy in these patients differs from that of the usual patient with Coats's disease. It is tempting to suspect that some feature of long standing retinitis pigmentosa has led to the development of this unusual peripheral vasculopathy.

While Geltzer and Berson (1969) have shown angiographically that the retinal macrocirculation of younger retinitis pigmentosa patients is normal, Best et al. (1972) have demonstrated delayed transit times and reversals of the relative opening pressures in choroidal and retinal circulations in some older retinitis pigmentosa patients. The minimum age at which Best was able to demonstrate retinal circulatory abnormality was 17 years. This corresponds well with the age of the youngest patients in our series, 16 years. The circulatory changes associated with retinitis pigmentosa may produce peripheral capillary closure, secondary shunting and telangiectasia and vascular leakage. The exudative

TABLE I

Case	Age	Sex	Race	Bilateral	Reference
1	22	M	W	Yes	Our case
2	39	F	W	Yes	Morgan & Crawford (1968)
3	16	F	W	Yes	Morgan & Crawford (1968)
4	35	M	W	Yes	Schmidt & Faulborn (1970)
5	25	F	W	Yes	Schmidt & Faulborn (1970)
6	16	F	W	*	Zamorani (1956)
7	22	F	W	No	Egerer et al. (1974)[#]

*A dense cataract prevented observation of one eye.

[#]Details of this case were kindly supplied by Dr. Tasman

detachment produced by such leakage results in the Coats-like syndrome. This hypothesis would explain the absence of the association in children, the lack of a sex predilection and the generally bilateral occurrence. Since the etiology of these cases seems to differ from that of the usual Coats's disease patient, the response to treatment may also differ. Indeed, of the 18 patients treated by Egerer et al. (1974), only three patients were classified as failures and one of these three had retinitis pigmentosa. The cryosurgical treatment in our case did seem to be of benefit, but one year following treatment, exudate was still present.

SUMMARY

Retinitis pigmentosa is occasionally associated with a vasculopathy of the Coats type. Although the clinical appearance of the vasculopathy is similar to that seen in the usual patient with Coats's disease, cases associated with retinitis pigmentosa are usually bilateral, equally common in females, and are not seen in childhood. These findings suggest a different etiological process.

We speculate that the etiology in such cases may be related to the vascular narrowing and slower circulation known to occur in some retinitis pigmentosa patients.

REFERENCES

Best, M., Toyofuku, H., and Galin, M. (1972) Ocular hemodynamics in retinitis pigmentosa. *Arch. Ophthal.* 88:123-130.

Egerer, I., Tasman, W., and Tomer, T. L. (1974) Coats's disease. *Arch. Ophthal.* 92:109-112.

Geltzer, A. I. and Berson, E. L. (1969) Fluorescein angiography of hereditary retinal degeneration. *Arch. Ophthal.* 81:776-782.

Morgan, W. E., III and Crawford, J. B. (1968) Retinitis pigmentosa and Coats's disease. *Arch. Ophthal.* 79:146-149.

Schmidt, D. and Faulborn, J. (1970) Retinopathia pigmentosa mit Coats-Syndrom. *Klin. Monatsbl. Augenheilk.* 157:643-652.

Wise, G. N., Dollery, C. T., and Henkind, P. (1971) "The Retinal Circulation," Harper and Row, New York, p. 256.

Zamorani, G. (1956) Una rara associatione di retinite di Coats con retinite pigmentosa. *Giornali Italiano di oftalmologica* 9(3): 429-443.

ACKNOWLEDGEMENTS

The authors wish to express their gratitude to Dr. Donald R. Bergsma for obtaining one of the references and to Dr. Myron L. Wolbarsht for his assistance with the figure and references.

DISCUSSION OF THE PAPER

DR. LATIES: The results with the amino acid analysis are interesting. You are about the only one who has tested for them. I don't know if all of you appreciate the clinical meaning of amino acids and retinopathy. There is now some evidence that certain types of retinitis pigmentosa, apparently secondary in nature, have amino acid difficulties or other metabolic abnormalities. Dr. Young, this morning, gave a list of the conditions that we look toward. The one that is best described by both Tackey and McCullough is gyrate atrophy, in which ornithine is abnormal.

DR. LATIES: Dr. Wadsworth, would you like to make any comments on the affinity for the blood vessel for pigment? There is a great deal of pigment around the blood vessel.

DR. WADSWORTH: I just don't know what to say about it.

DR. WEINSTEIN: I have a question about the decreased visual acuity and response to cryotherapy. Was there lipid in the macular area? How do you explain the improvement?

DR. WADSWORTH: There was some edema in the posterior pole associated with this Coats-like proteinaceous material in the periphery and posterior pole, and the retina did flatten considerably, and this Coats-like process was much improved. I explain the improvement of vision on that situation.

TRACE METALS IN A FAMILY WITH SEX-LINKED RETINITIS PIGMENTOSA

James Bastek*, John Bogden#, Alfonse Cinotti*,
William TenHove+, George Stephens*,
Michael Markopoulos*, and James Charles*

Department of Ophthalmology*
Department of Preventive Medicine#
Department of Medicine+

New Jersey Medical School (CMDNJ)
Newark, New Jersey 07103

INTRODUCTION

Our review of the literature on trace metals (Hughes and Coogan, 1974; Halsted and Smith, 1974; Niklowitz and Yeager, 1973; Henkin and Smith, 1972; Figueroa et al., 1971; Sorsby and Harding, 1962) suggested the possibility of a previously unsuspected relationship between body burdens of trace metals and retinitis pigmentosa (RP). The metals chosen for investigation were cadmium, lead, zinc, and copper. Lead values were examined because animal studies (Hughes and Coogan, 1974) have shown that tapetoretinal degeneration can be induced in rabbits by treatment with lead acetate. Lead is believed to exert its toxic effects on the central nervous system by replacing neural copper and zinc (Niklowitz and Yeager, 1973). Zinc and copper were studied because the general chelating agent, dithizone, induces tapetoretinal degeneration in experimental animals (Grant, 1974). In cirrhosis, plasma zinc levels are reduced, and there is speculation (Halsted and Smith, 1974) that low levels of zinc interfere with vitamin A therapy in night blindness. In hepatitis patients there is a positive correlation between zinc and retinol binding protein (Henkin and Smith, 1972). Decoloration of the tapetum lucidum of the dog eye was produced by a single oral 1600 mg/kg dose of ethambutol (Figueroa et al., 1971). This effect was correlated with a decrease of the zinc concentration of the tissue. Cadmium levels were determined, since cadmium binds with sulfur and inhibition of sulfhydryl groups may cause retinotoxic effects (Sorsby and Harding, 1962).

43

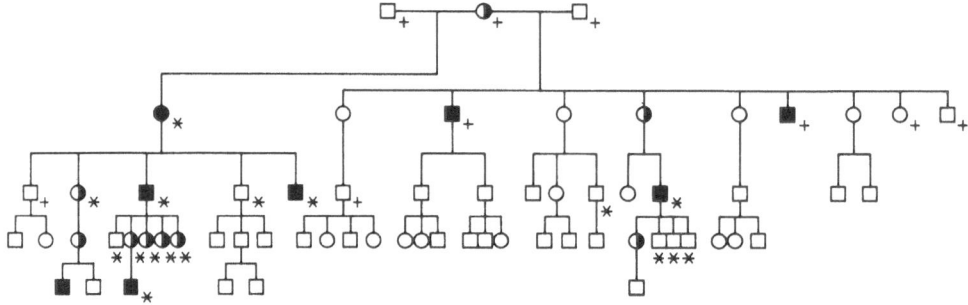

FIGURE 1. Pedigree of the family studied with sex-linked retinitis
   pigmentosa. Those who had blood drawn for the study are indicated with an asterisk (*).

Retinitis pigmentosa, which may be acquired or produced by
various types of hereditary transmission, may be a common denomina-
tor manifestation of different disease processes. Therefore, it
was decided that each type of RP should first be studied within
each subcategory. Sex-linked RP is a convenient and interesting
type to study because controls, carriers, and victims can be selected from within one family. We studied these three groups within
one family with a history of sex-linked RP.

METHODS

The family studied has had eight cases of RP spread over four
generations. Two victims are deceased. The family members from
whom blood was drawn are indicated with an asterisk in Fig. 1.
These were the only family members available for the study: six
controls, five carriers, and five RP patients. Controls were
family members who did not have the disease and were not carriers.
Carriers were female daughters of an RP victim or were the mothers
or grandmothers of RP victims. The diagnosis of RP in the victims
was confirmed by ERG, EOG, dark adaptation, and visual fields.

The collection of samples followed standardized literature
methods (Anand *et al.*, 1975). Fasting early morning (7:30 - 9:30

WHOLE BLOOD LEAD (μg/100ml)		PLASMA COPPER (μg/100ml)		PLASMA ZINC (μg/100ml)		ZINC/COPPER RATIO	
CONTROLS							
17		88		100		1.14	
14		86		112		1.30	
12	18 ±3.9	72	81 ±6.5	86	92 ±12.0	1.19	1.14 ±0.10
21	AVG ±SD	74	AVG ±SD	80	AVG ±SD	1.08	AVG ±SD
19		84		84		1.00	
22		80		88		1.10	
CARRIERS							
10		96		114		1.19	
18	15 ±4.1	86	90 ±6.9	106	115 ±13.8	1.23	1.28 ±0.19
12	AVG ±SD	80	AVG ±SD	118	AVG ±SD	1.48	AVG ±SD
14		96		100		1.04	
20		92		136		1.48	
RP'S							
29		114		100		0.88	
19	20 ±7.1	82	111 ±21.6	68	92 ±15.1	0.83	0.83 ±0.08
20	AVG ±SD	136	AVG ±SD	94	AVG ±SD	0.69	AVG ±SD
21		126		108		0.86	
9		98		88		0.90	

FIGURE 2. Summary of whole blood lead, plasma copper and plasma zinc levels from family members. A zinc/copper ratio was calculated for each family member. Within each group an average (AVG) was calculated along with the standard deviation (SD).

a.m.) samples were obtained. Precautions were taken to avoid contamination by the use of plastic syringes instead of vacutainers and the use of pre-rinsed heparinized plastic tubes to transport and store the samples. Half of the sample was centrifuged to obtain plasma to determine the copper and zinc concentrations. The remaining whole blood was used to determine the cadmium and lead concentrations. All of the samples were analyzed by atomic absorption spectrophotometry. The analyses were performed by using previously reported techniques (Westerlund-Helmerson, 1970; Hessel, 1968; Parker *et al.*, 1967; Perkin-Elmer, 1971). One RP victim had a lymphoma, but none of the other subjects in the study had any concurrent or recent illness. None of the females was taking oral contraceptives, and none was pregnant.

RESULTS

Figure 2 lists the results, and Figs. 3 and 4 display the plasma copper and zinc values more graphically. All of the cadmium concentrations were less than 1.0 μg%. Similarly, lead concentrations did not differ significantly among the groups.

The average concentration of plasma copper increased progressively from controls (81±6.5) to carriers (90±6.9) to victims (111±21.6). The RP group had significantly higher plasma copper levels ($p < 0.01$, t-test) than did the control group. The carrier group also had significantly higher plasma copper levels ($p < 0.05$, t-test) than did the control group. The normal range of plasma copper concentration is from 60 to 150 μg% for the method we employed.

Plasma zinc concentrations were found to be significantly higher ($p < 0.05$, t-test) in the carrier group (115±13.8) than in either the control group (92±12.0) or the RP group (92±15.1). The mean plasma zinc concentration for the carrier group was 115 μg%.

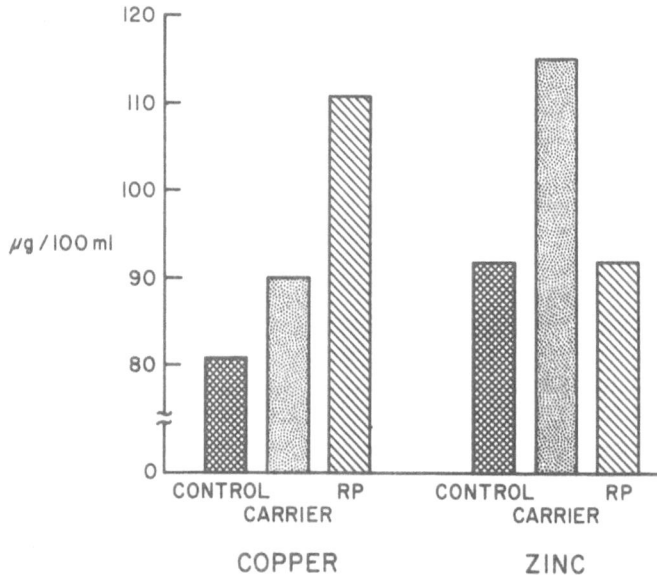

FIGURE 3. Summary of average plasma copper and average plasma/zinc concentrations within each group within the family.

The normal range of plasma zinc concentration is from 55 to 115 µg%
for the method we employed. Therefore, the mean plasma zinc concentration for the carrier group was at the upper limit of normal.

The ratio of plasma zinc to copper was calculated. For all of
the carriers and controls, this value was greater than 1.0. However, for all those in the RP group, this value was less than 1.0.
The ratios within the RP group (0.83±0.08) were significantly
lower than those in the carrier group (1.28±0.19) or those in the
control group (1.14±0.10). These differences were both statistically significant ($p < 0.01$, t-test).

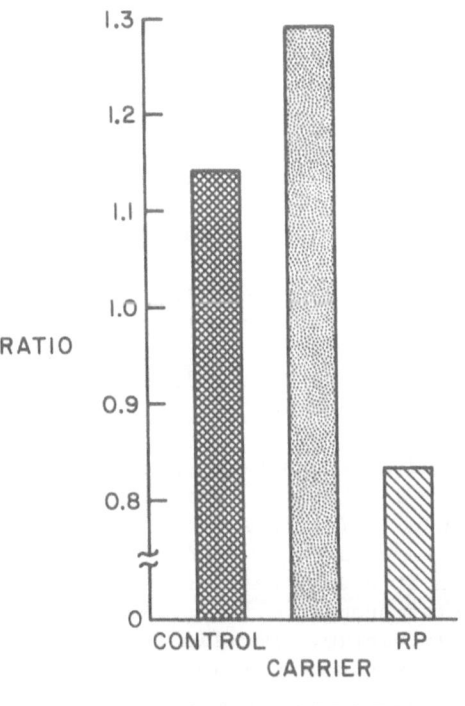

FIGURE 4. Summary of the average plasma zinc/plasma copper ratio
within each group within the family.

DISCUSSION

Plasma zinc concentrations decrease and plasma copper concentrations increase in a number of stress states, but the mechanism
for these changes in copper and zinc has not been established.
The ratio of plasma concentrations of zinc to copper is altered in
some diseases.   It is depressed in patients with chronic liver
infections, liver diseases, lymphoma, pernicious anemia and leukemia (Delves *et al*., 1973; Underwood, 1971; Rosner and Gorfien,
1968).   In leukemia the ratio of these two metals has been used to
monitor patient response during treatment (Delves *et al*., 1973).

These findings may be of diagnostic significance. One of the
victims is a 5 year old male, currently asymptomatic. His ratio of
plasma zinc to copper is less than 1.0, as is true of the other RP
victims in the family. In attempting to identify a sex-linked
carrier, higher levels of zinc may lend supporting evidence to any
ERG or visual abnormalities.

One of the RP victims in the family was a manifesting hetero-
zygote. In late life she began to display symptoms of the disease
and several years ago was diagnosed as having RP. At that time,
however, an ERG was not done. About one and one-half years ago,
she was found to have lymphoma, a disease known to lower plasma
zinc levels. During this study, the diagnosis of RP was confirmed
by means of an ERG, EOG, and dark adaptation tests. The group of
heterozygous carriers had plasma zinc levels which averaged at the
upper limit of normal. If this higher level of zinc is in some
way protective against RP for the carriers, then a chronic disease
or condition which depressed plasma zinc levels for an extended
period of time may be involved in transforming nonmanifesting
heterozygous carriers into manifesting heterozygotes. One condition which depresses plasma zinc levels is the use of oral
contraceptives (Halsted and Smith, 1970). Monitoring of sex-linked
carriers on oral contraceptives may be informative.

Some sex-linked carriers have been reported to have abnormalities in ERG, dark adaptation, and visual fields (Jay and Bird,
1973; Bird and Hyman, 1972; Berson *et al*., 1969). There exists the
possibility that some carriers have a milder form of RP. If that
is the case, then it seems reasonable to assume that they are bio-
chemically protected against the severe progression which befalls
the sex-linked male victim. Our findings suggest that zinc and/or
copper metabolism may somehow be involved in such a protection.

SUMMARY

Lead, cadmium, copper, and zinc levels were examined in RP
patients, carriers, and controls in a family with sex-linked RP.

The mean plasma copper concentration was significantly higher in the RP patients and carriers than in the controls. The mean plasma zinc concentration was significantly higher in the carriers than in the RP victims or controls. The mean plasma zinc/copper ratio was significantly lower in the RP victims than in the controls or carriers. These findings may help explain the onset of RP in some sex-linked carriers and may be of diagnostic value.

REFERENCES

Anand, V. D., White, J. M., and Nino, H. V. (1975) Some aspects of specimen collection and stability in trace element analysis of body fluids. *Clin. Chem.* 21:595-602.

Bird, A. C., and Hyman, V. (1972) Detection of heterozygotes in families with X-linked pigmentary retinopathy by measurement of retinal rhodopsin concentration. *Trans. Ophthal. Soc. UK* 92:221-229.

Berson, E. L., Gouras, P., Gunkel, R. D., and Myrianthopoulos, N. C. (1969) Rod and cone responses in sex-linked retinitis pigmentosa. *Arch. Ophthal.* 81:215-225.

Delves, H. T., Alexander, F. W., and Lay, H. (1973) Copper and zinc concentration in the plasma of leukemic children. *Brit. J. Haematol.* 24:525-531.

Figueroa, R., Weiss, H., Smith, J. C., Jr., Hackley, B. M., McBean, L. D., Swassing, C. R., and Halsted, J. A. (1971) Effect of ethambutol on the ocular zinc concentration in dogs. *Amer. Rev. Resp. Dis.* 104:592-594.

Grant, W. M. (1974) "Toxicology of the Eye" (ed. 2), p. 42, Charles C Thomas, Springfield, Illinois.

Halsted, J. A., and Smith, J. C., Jr. (1974) Night blindness and chronic liver disease. *Gastroenterology* 67:193-194.

Halsted, J. A., and Smith, J. C., Jr. (1970) Plasma-zinc in health and disease. *Lancet* 1(7642):322-324.

Henkin, R. J., and Smith, F. R. (1972) Zinc and copper metabolism in acute viral hepatitis. *Amer. J. Med. Sci.* 264:401-409.

Hessel, D. W. (1968) A simple and rapid quantitative determination of lead in blood. *Atomic Absorption Newsletter* 7:55-56.

Hughes, W. F., and Coogan, P. S. (1974) Pathology of the pigment epithelium and retina in rabbits poisoned with lead. *Amer. J. Path.* 77:237-254.

Jay, B., and Bird, A. (1973) X-linked retinitis pigmentosa. *Trans. Amer. Acad. Ophthal.* 77:641-651.

Niklowitz, W. J., and Yeater, D. W. (1973) Interference of lead with essential brain tissue. Copper, iron and zinc as main determinant in experimental tetraethyl lead. *Life Science* 13:897-305.

Parker, M. M., Humoller, F. L., and Mahler, D. J. (1967) Determination of copper and zinc in biological material. *Clin. Chem.* 13:40-48.

Perkin-Elmer Corporation (1971) Clinical Methods for Atomic Absorption Spectroscopy. Norwalk, Connecticut, pp. Cu 1,1 and Zn 1,1.

Rosner, F., and Gorfien, P. C. (1968) Erythrocyte and plasma zinc and magnesium levels in health and disease. *J. Lab. Clin. Med.* 72:213-219.

Sorsby, A., and Harding, R. (1962) Experimental degeneration of the retina--X. *Vis. Res.* 2:327-330.

Underwood, E. J. (1971) "Trace Metals in Human and Animal Nutrition," Chapter 8, Academic Press, New York.

Westerlund-Helmerson, V. (1970) Determination of lead and cadmium in blood by a modification of the Hessel Method. *Atomic Absorption Newsletter* 9:133-134.

OCULAR CHANGES IN LAURENCE MOON BARDET BIEDL SYNDROME: A CLINICAL

AND HISTOPATHOLOGIC STUDY OF A CASE

Moshe Lahav, Daniel M. Albert, Ned Buyukmihci,
Lee Jampol, Edward B. McLean*, Rufus Howard,
and Joseph Craft

Department of Ophthalmology and Visual Science
Yale University School of Medicine
333 Cedar Street
New Haven, Connecticut   06510

Department of Ophthalmology*
University of Washington
Seattle, Washington

INTRODUCTION

The Laurence Moon Bardet Biedl Syndrome (LMBBS) is a rare
familial disorder classically characterized by five major findings:
mental retardation, obesity, polydactyly, hypogonadism, and retinitis pigmentosa.   This report describes the clinical and light and
electron microscopic ocular changes in an 18 year old male patient
with this syndrome.

CASE REPORT

The patient, a white male, was born October 15, 1954, following a full term pregnancy complicated by mild toxemia.   At birth he
weighed 4.2 kg and was 59 cm long.   The findings on physical examination were within normal limits.   Review of the family history
revealed that three maternal uncles had alcaptonuria and died
during childhood or adolescence.   There was no other family incidence of LMBBS and no visual defects were known in other family
members.   The patient's mother and his two older sisters were in
good health; the father had adult onset diabetes mellitus and
required insulin therapy.   The patient had bilateral inguinal

51

herniorrhaphies at 10 months of age. He remained short in stature, was obese and exhibited excessive thirst from infancy.

The patient was examined initially at the Yale New Haven Hospital in November, 1966, when he was 12 years of age. He was below the third percentile in height (138 cm) and greater than the 97th percentile in weight (64.3 kg). He appeared to be mentally retarded. Additional physical findings included stubby hands and feet, and ill-defined knuckles (Fig. 1). He had a small penis, first degree hypospadias and non-palpable gonads. His blood pressure was 190/120. Radiograms of the hands and feet showed shortening of the phalanges, metacarpals and metatarsals, but no polydactyly. Dorsal scoliosis and an enlarged skull without signs of increased cerebrospinal fluid pressure were demonstrated. The serum calcium was 9.1 mg/100 ml and the serum phosphorus 4.1 mg/100 ml. The serum proteins were normal at that time. A definitive diagnosis was not established. Following treatment with chorionic gonadotrophins and testosterone, the patient showed increased penis size but no apparent testicular maturation. Pubic hair developed and his voice deepened.

Significant renal disease first became apparent in 1971. His blood urea nitrogen was 64 mg% and his creatinine clearance rate was 15 cc per minute. The urine osmolarity was found to be 233 osmoles and did not change following administration of intramuscular vasopressin. This was interpreted as indicating nephrogenic diabetes incipidus. An intravenous pyelogram revealed shrunken kidneys. The findings on cystography were normal. In the final months his blood pressure was intermittently elevated, and he demonstrated tetany on several occasions. His renal disease progressed, and he died at the age of 18 years with terminal uremia.

The following laboratory tests were carried out and the results were normal: white blood count and differential; hemoglobin; protein bound iodine, T_3 and T_4; fluorescent treponema antibody-absorbed test; buccal smear; radiograms of the sella tursica and optic foramina; bone age evaluation; karyotyping by the Q-banding technique; and audiology.

Eye Examination

The patient's first recorded visual acuity was in 1963 at age 8 years and was 20/40 in each eye. Other details of this examination are not known.

At 13 years of age he was seen at the Yale New Haven eye clinic for evaluation of symptoms of night blindness. His best corrected visual acuity was 20/80 in each eye. Refraction revealed moderate myopic astigmatism in each eye. He had occasional fine

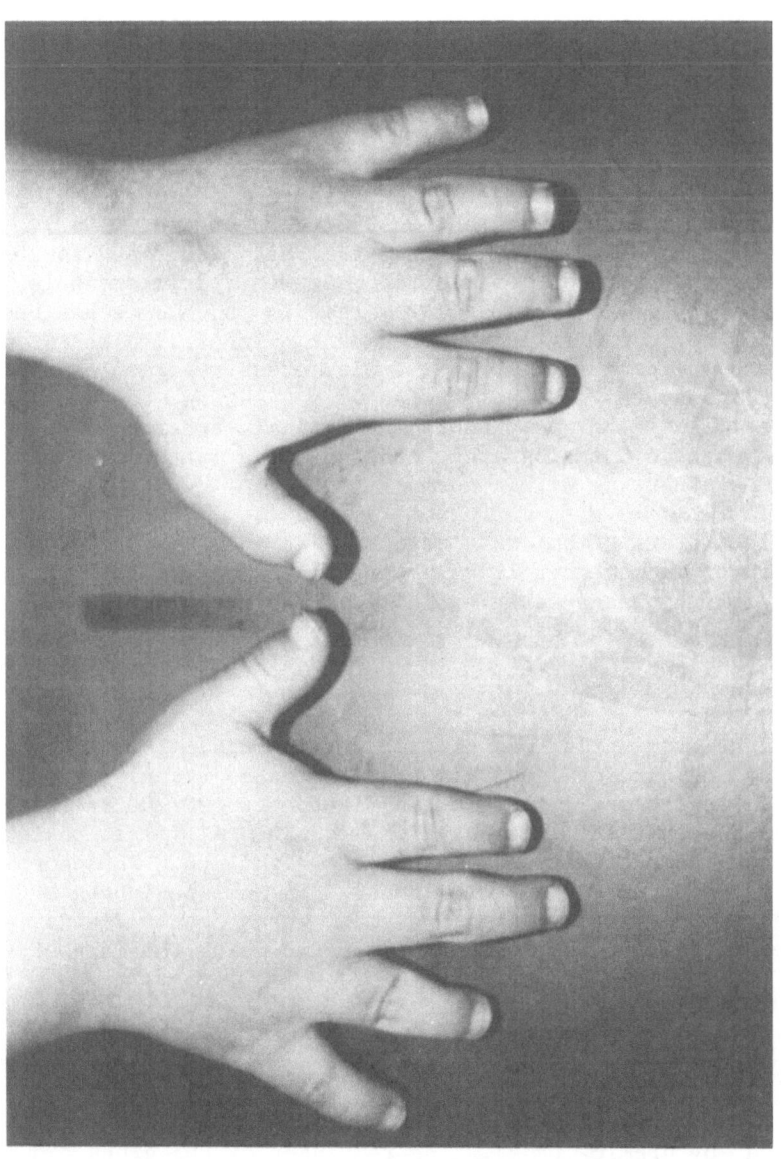

FIGURE 1. Note the stubby phalanges and ill-defined knuckles.

rotary and vertical jerk movements bilaterally. The anterior segments were unremarkable and the intraocular pressures within normal
limits. There was pallor to both optic discs. A fine granular
appearance of the retinal pigment was present in the posterior pole
and periphery. The peripheral fields were not reliable due to poor
fixation, but appeared to be constricted to approximately 5-10°
using the largest and brightest test objects in each eye. The
patient was unable to correctly interpret a single Ishihara or
Hardy Rand Rittler (HRR) color plate.

Over the following two years his eyes were examined at six
month intervals. An alternating exotropia of 12 prism diopters
(PD) was noted when the patient was 15 years of age (1970). His
best corrected visual acuity at this time had decreased to 20/100
in each eye. On retinal examination, a peripapillary halo was
noted in the left eye. The macular areas in both eyes had become
granular and no foveal reflex was evident (Fig. 2). With a fundus
contact lens, examination of the macular areas revealed an irregular wrinkling of the retinal surface, suggesting contraction of
the internal limiting membrane. The retinal arterioles appeared
narrow. Fluorescein angiography confirmed the arteriolar narrowing, but was otherwise within normal limits.

An electroretinogram was performed at New York University
Medical Center in November 1970, by Dr. Ronald Carr. Both photopic
and scotopic responses were extinct by the techniques used. The
Farnsworth Panel D-15 test indicated essentially normal color
placement ability, although he again missed HRR and Ishihara color
plates.

The last examination was carried out in July, 1973, when the
patient was 18 years of age. His best corrected visual acuity was
now count fingers at 1 foot in the right eye; 20/200 in the left
eye. The alternating exotropia was 20 PD. A small posterior
subcapsular cataract was present in the right eye. The choroidal
pattern was prominent in both fundi. In the periphery of the
retinas some scattered pigment clumps were seen. Fields were
restricted to 3-5° on the Goldmann perimeter using the largest test
objects.

Autopsy Findings

The patient was 155 cm tall and weighed 81.8 kg. The skin
was covered by uremic frost. The remainder of the gross examination conformed to the physical findings previously described,
including the obesity and hypogonadism. Forty cubic centimeters
of serous fluid was present in the thoracic cavity. Positive gross
and microscopic findings are given in Table I. The diagnosis of
LMBBS was confirmed.

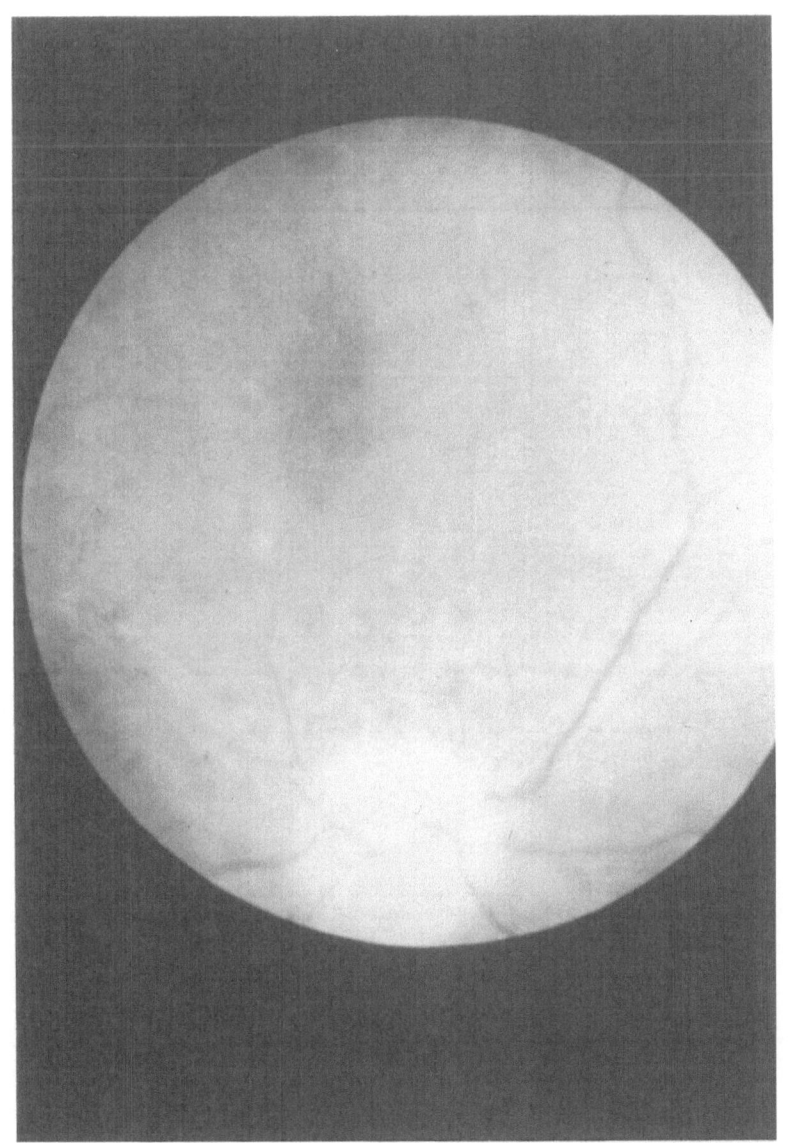

FIGURE 2. Fundus photograph O.S. Note lack of foveal reflex and granular appearance to macula.

TABLE I

AUTOPSY FINDINGS

Brain

Gross Examination	Microscopic Examination
Some cortical atrophy was considered to be present; the ventricular system was moderately dilated; some gyri were poorly separated (especially frontoparietal).	Optic chiasm: no significant abnormality; fibers are well myelinated.
	Lateral geniculate body: intact and normal.
	Third ventricle: ependymal lining contained many proliferations of neuroglia consistent with an old granular ependymitis.
	Sections of cortex, hippocampus, thalamus, basal ganglion, pons, cerebrum essentially normal. There was a mild decrease of neurons in inferior olive.

Thyroid

Right and left lobes were small and most of the parenchyma was in the isthmus.	Epithelium was hypoplastic.

Kidneys

Small, shrunken, and scarred (R, 28 gm; L, 48 gm); hydronephrosis and multiple retention cysts were present bilaterally; both renal arteries were small.	The glomeruli were dysplastic. There was loss of some tubules and dilatation of others.

Ureters	Dilated without obstruction.
Bladder	Diverticulum present.
Testis	Only a single undescended testicle was identified. A reduced number of Leydig interstitial cells. The walls of the seminiferous tubules were fibrotic. No mature spermatozoa were seen.
Skeletal	Mild osteoporosis was present with hypoplastic marrow. Evidence of maturational development of most bone marrow elements.
Vascular	Large and medium vessels were thin walled with narrow lumens.

EYE PATHOLOGY

Materials and Methods

Light microscopy. The eyes were enucleated approximately four hours after death, fixed in 10% buffered formalin, dehydrated and embedded in paraffin. Eight micrometer pupil-optic nerve sections were cut from each eye. Staining procedures included: Harris hematoxylin and eosin (H & E), periodic acid Schiff (PAS), AFIP lipofuscin stain (Luna, 1968), Putt's method for acid fast orga- nisms, luxol fast blue for phospholipids, osmium tetraoxide 1% and Fontana-Masson silver stain for argentaffin granules. The sections were examined by conventional (tungsten light) microscopy and by ultraviolet fluorescent and polarizing light microscopy. Addi- tional sections were cut from the formalin fixed wet tissue and stained with the oil red-0 technique.

Control studies. Three globes were processed in an identical manner and served as control: (a) a clinically and histologically normal globe from a four year old Caucasian female who died of tracheal stenosis; (b) a globe from a 48 year old Caucasian female containing a malignant melanoma of the posterior choroid (spindle B cell type); and (c) an eye from an 88 year old Caucasian male with a clinical history and findings of retinitis pigmentosa since childhood, who died from arteriosclerotic heart disease.

Electron microscopy. The macular area of the LMBBS left eye was dissected out of the paraffin block and processed for electron microscopy in a manner previously described (Tso, 1970). Ultrathin sections were cut on the LKB Ultratome II and observed with the Siemens Elmiskop I.

Results

Gross examination. Both eyes of the LMBBS patient had a simi- lar appearance. The right globe was intact and measured 23 x 24 x 24 mm with 9 mm of optic nerve attached. The cornea measured 11 x 11 mm; the pupil was 5 mm in diameter and round. The eye was opened in the horizontal meridian. The anterior segment was within normal limits except for posterior cortical lenticular opacities. The vitreous was liquid and clear and mostly lost in sectioning. The neural retina appeared attached. The macular area was puckered and appeared granular. No fovea centralis was evident. Scattered pigmented clumps were present at the equator, particularly inferi- orly. The choroidal pattern was strikingly prominent (Figs. 3a, 3b). The sclera was thinned in the equatorial region. The left eye was essentially similar, except for the presence of a slightly raised, round, dark gray lesion about three-quarters of the disc diameter in size in the superior calotte at the equator.

Microscopic examination. The histologic appearance of both eyes is similar except with regard to the macular areas. The cornea, anterior chamber, and iris are within normal limits. The scleral spur is poorly developed and the ciliary muscle inserts into the trabecular meshwork (Fig. 4). The lens shows posterior migration of epithelial cells, with occasional absence of lens epithelium anteriorly. Vacuolization and fragmentation of cortical lens fibers are seen in the anterior and posterior cortex (Fig. 5). Some liquified vitreous remains. The retina shows thinning of all layers (Figs. 6a, 6b) with narrowed vessels and the presence of pigment laden macrophages. Cystoid spaces are present in the nerve fiber layer. The ganglion cells are decreased in number with the relatively thick layer of ganglion cells showing pyknotic changes in the macular area. The inner nuclear layer in some areas is in close proximity to the outer nuclear layer (Fig. 7). Only short thickened remnants of the photoreceptors are seen beyond the external limiting membrane. In the macular area of the left eye the photoreceptor cell layer is represented by a single layer of cuboidal cells bounded by an external limiting membrane (Fig. 8). The external plexiform layer is edematous in this area; internal to this are multilayered bipolar and ganglion cells. The internal limiting membrane is wrinkled in the macular area. The retinal pigment epithelium (RPE) appears hypopigmented posteriorly, with occasional intracytoplasmic granules (Fig. 9). At the equator the pigment epithelium is flattened and shows patchy, atrophic and hypertrophic areas. The choroid is thin and the choriocapillaris shows atrophy posteriorly. Irregular aggregates of heavily pigmented choroidal melanocytes are seen. The pigmented lesion seen grossly at the superior equator of the left eye appears to be hyperplastic pigmented epithelium internal to a plaque-like mass of epithelioid cells (Fig. 10). The optic nerve is atrophic, and the sclera shows thinning in the equatorial region (Fig. 11).

Diagnosis

1. Abnormality of the neural retina in both eyes with decreased numbers of ganglion cells, thinning of the nerve fiber, bipolar and photoreceptor cell layers with widespread absence of photoreceptor cell elements.

2. Atrophy and hypertrophy of the retinal pigment epithelium with evidence of intraretinal migration of pigmented cells.

3. Nevus-like clumping of the choroidal melanocytes, atrophy of the choriocapillaris.

4. Optic atrophy.

5. Plaque-like proliferations of retinal pigment epithelium at the
   superior equator of the left eye.

6. Incomplete cleavage of the chamber angle.

7. Early cataracts.

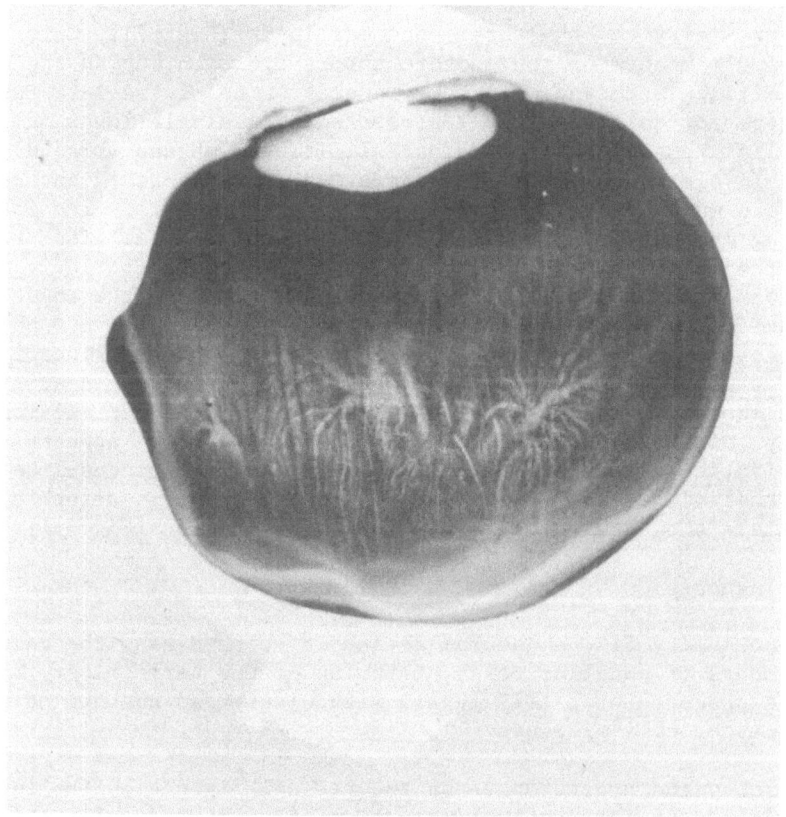

FIGURE 3a. Gross photograph of opened left globe to show prominent
   choroidal pattern.

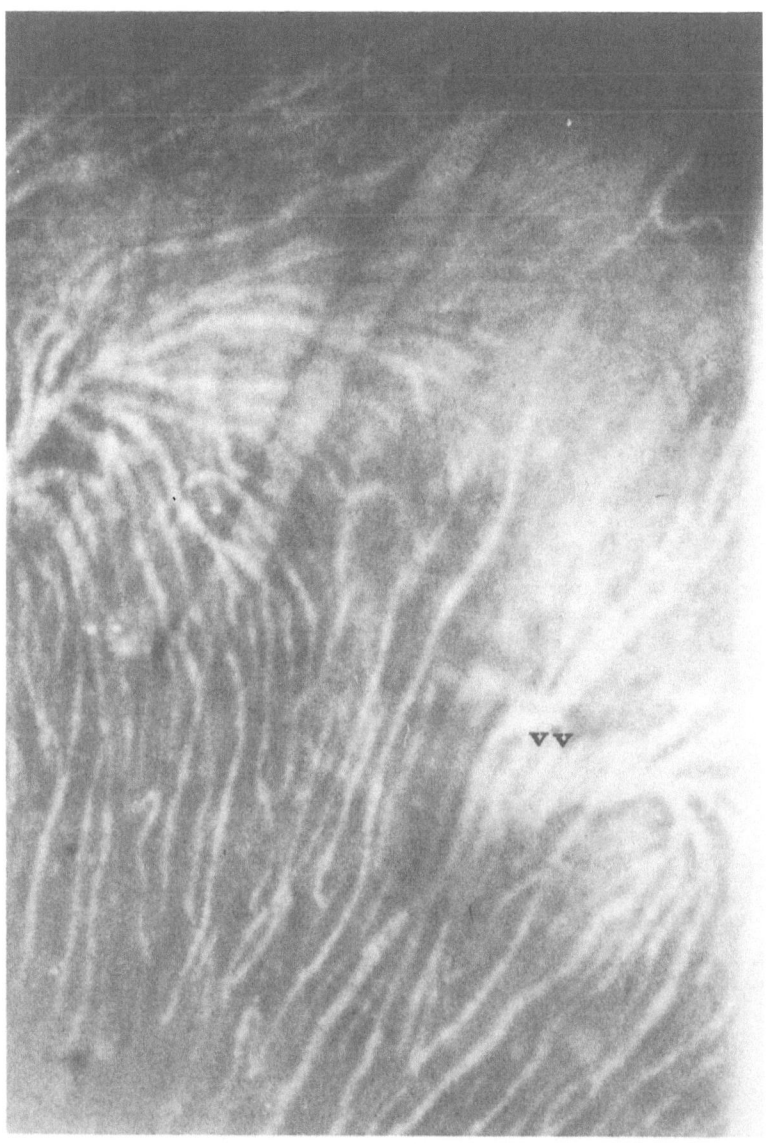

FIGURE *3b*. Higher magnification of choroidal area to show marked prominence of the vortex veins (VV) and other choroidal vessels.

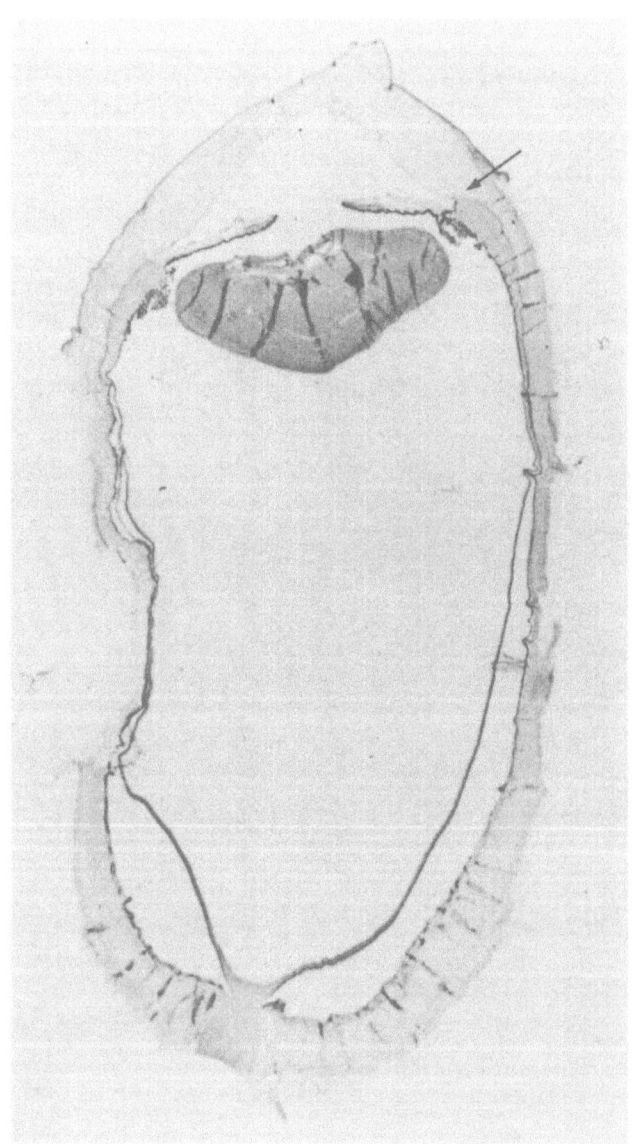

FIGURE 4. Abnormal insertion of the ciliary body muscle into the
      trabecular meshwork (arrow). Both eyes were similar in appear-
      ance. (H & E x200)

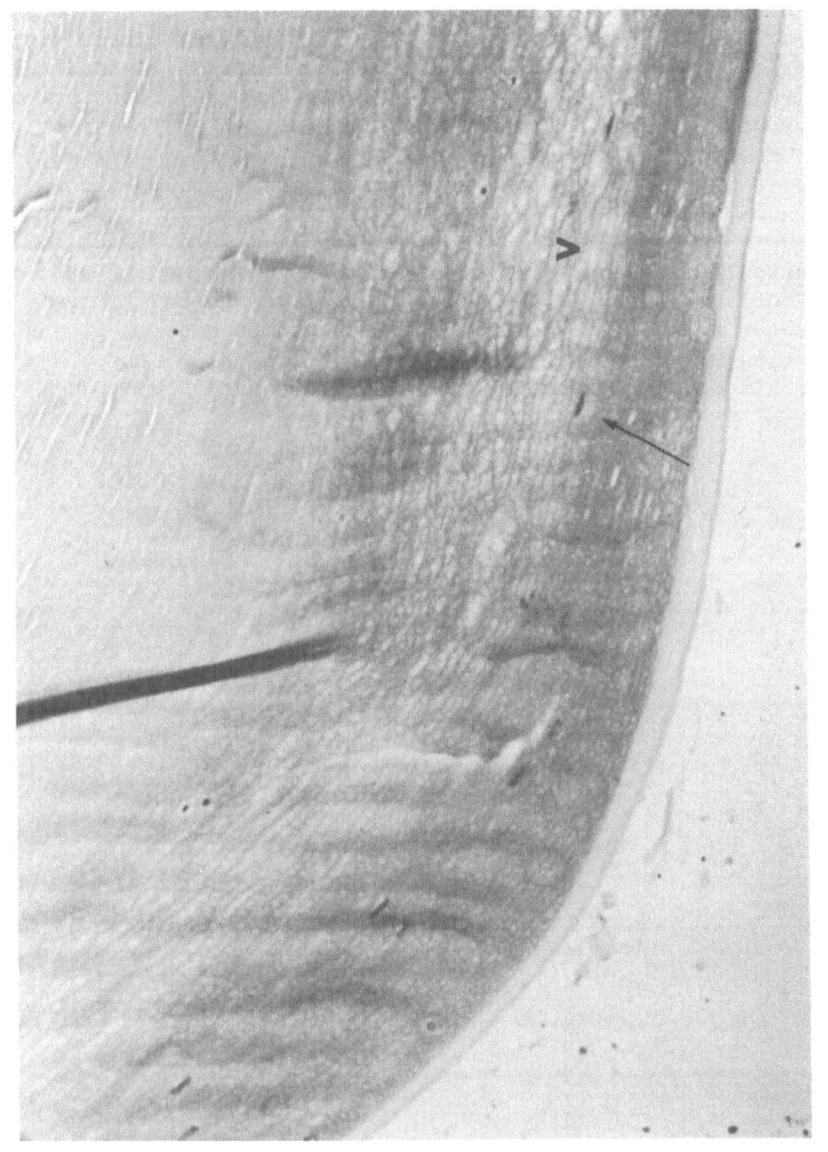

FIGURE 5. Posterior migration of nuclei (arrow) and minimal vacuolization of the posterior cortical lens fibers (V). (H & E x200)

Special stains. In the LMBBS patient, the granules which were
seen in the pigment epithelium stained well with the oil red-0
technique. Decreased numbers of granules were seen with lipofuscin
stains as compared to all of the "control" eyes examined. In addition, no staining with acid fast or luxol fast blue stains could be
identified. The PAS reaction gave only minimal identifiable stain.
Only part of the granules within the intraretinal pigmented cells
stained well with the lipofuscin stain and PAS reaction, but did
not react with the acid fast stain. Comparison of the various
staining characteristics of the RPE cells and the intraretinal
pigmented cells with the normal, retinitis pigmentosa, and malignant melanoma globes is given in Table II.

Electron microscopy. The cuboidal cells which constituted the
external nuclear layer in the left eye proved to be remnants of
photoreceptor cells. The cells were adherent to each other and to
Muller cells by means of terminal bars. External to these junc-
tions, small dilated sacs containing mitochondria were seen as

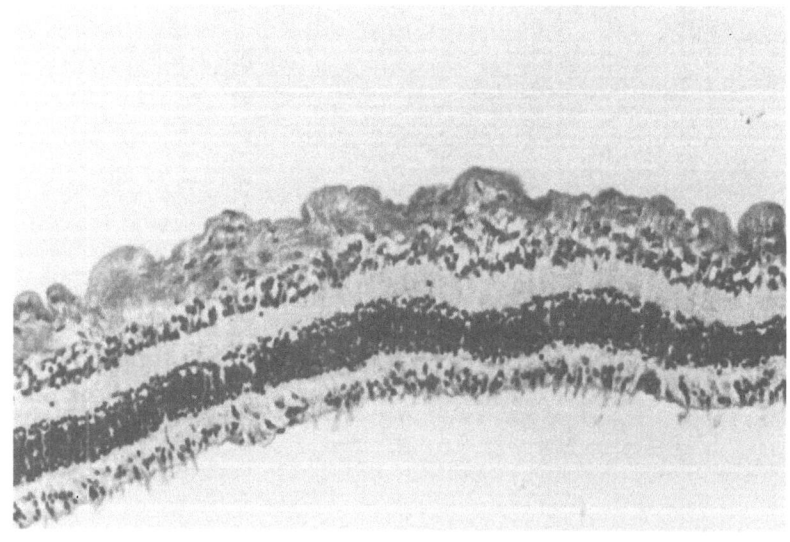

FIGURE 6a. Thinning of the retina in the left globe. Note the
narrowing of the outer nuclear layer. (H & E x100)

remnants of the photoreceptor inner segment. No outer segment
structures could be identified (Fig. 12). Basal bodies and root
filaments (Fig. 13), in addition to connecting cilia (Fig. 14),
were seen. The pigmented cells within the retina contained granules of melanin, compound melanin-lipofuscin granules and many
slightly osmiophilic vesicular bodies that probably represent lipid
granules other than mature lipofuscin (Figs. 15, 16). The exact
nature of these cells could not be determined with certainty.

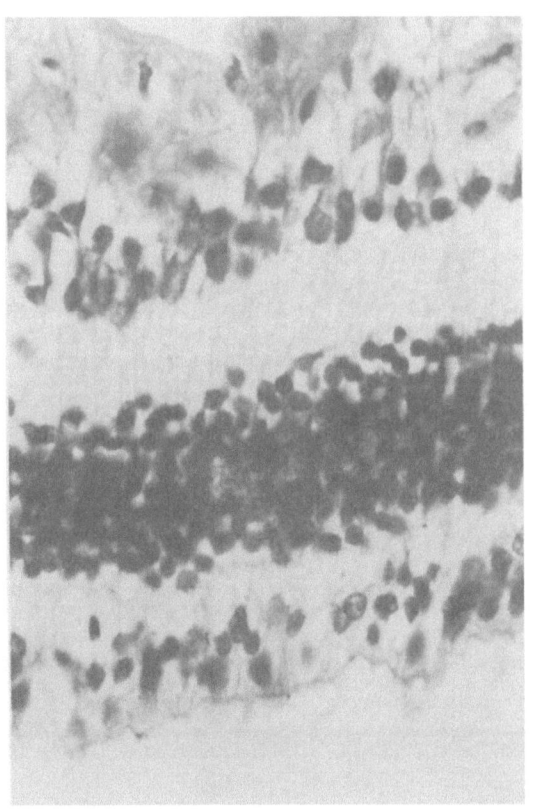

FIGURE 6b. Higher magnification of a portion of Fig. 6a. (H & E
     x400)

   Electron microscopy (EM) of the RPE showed pigment granules throughout the cytoplasm and most concentrated in the mid and apical portion of the cell extending into the areas normally in contact with the outer segment (Fig. 17). The nuclei which were confined to the basal portion of the cell seemed well preserved with diffuse chromatin (Fig. 17). Sparse rough endoplasmic reticulum was seen throughout the cytoplasm. Free ribosomes were identified as well as clusters of mitochondria at the base of the cells. The basement membrane of the RPE was well developed (Fig. 17).

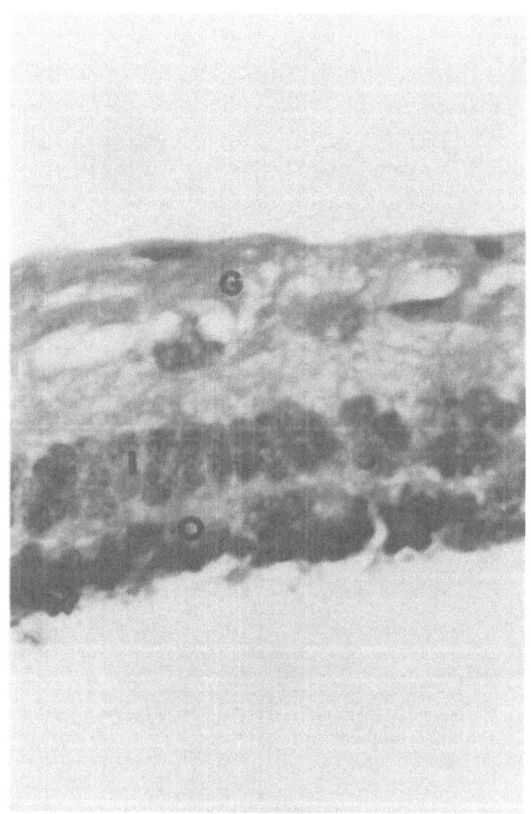

FIGURE 7. Retina from the equatorial region in the left eye. Note the absence of blood vessels, the loss of ganglion cells (G), and thinning of the inner (I) and outer (O) nuclear layers. (H & E x400)

In addition to the pigment granules in the RPE, premelanosomes and lipofuscin were observed as well. Overall, a greater proportion of developing pigment granules was present than mature granules. Rudiments of microvilli were seen at the cell surface of the RPE and cilia were often seen protruding from the RPE toward the outer segment region (Fig. 18).

The RPE cells were attached to each other by zonula occludens, zonula adherens, and desmosomes. The intercellular spaces were found to be well preserved (Fig. 19). Basal bodies, centrioles, and cross-striated rootlets of the cilia were also found in the RPE and showed no abnormal features (Fig. 20). Microtubules, smooth endoplasmic reticulum and other cytoplasmic organelles were not well preserved, presumably due to autolysis and initial formaldehyde fixation.

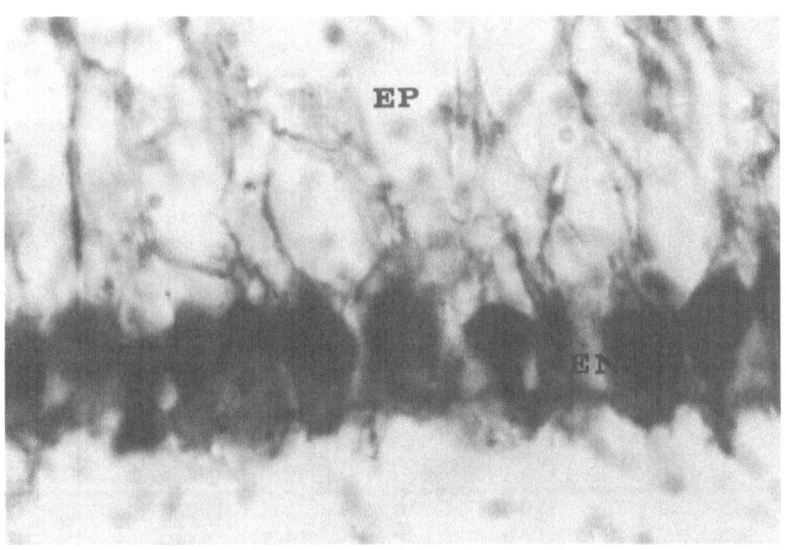

FIGURE 8. Macular area of the left globe. The external plexiform layer is edematous (EP) and the nuclear layer consists of a single row of nuclei (EN). (H & E x960)

LAHAV *et al.*

TABLE II

COMPARATIVE DIFFERENTIAL STAINING OF PIGMENTED CELLS

	Retinal Pigment Epithelium				Pigmented Cells Within the Retina		
	L–M–B[1]	RP[2]	MM[3]	NL[4]	L–M–B[1]	RP[2]	MM[3]
Oil Red O	+	+	+	+	+	+	+
Lipofuscin (AFIP)	±	+	+	+	+	±	±
Acid Fast	–	+	+	±	–	+	±
Luxol Fast Blue	–	–	–	–	–	–	–
Osmium	+	+	+	+	+	+	+
Fluorescence	+	+	+	+	+	+	+
PAS	±	±	+	±	+	–	+
Fontana Silver	+	+	+	+	+	±	+
Birefringence	–	–	–	–	–	–	–

[1]L–M–B Laurence–Moon–Biedl
[2]RP Retinitis Pigmentosa
[3]MM Malignant Melanoma
[4]NL Normal

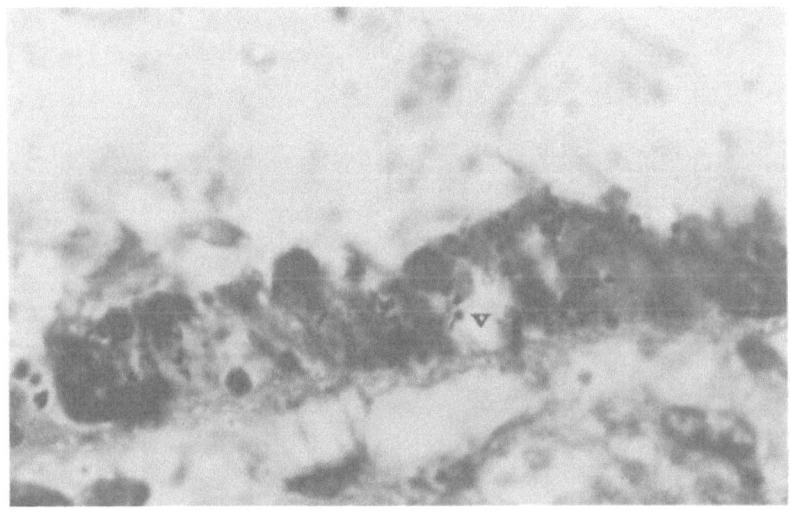

FIGURE 9. Patchy hypopigmentation of the pigment epithelium at the posterior pole in the left eye. Note the intraepithelial vacuolization (V) and the patchy atrophy of the choriocapillaris. (H & E x960)

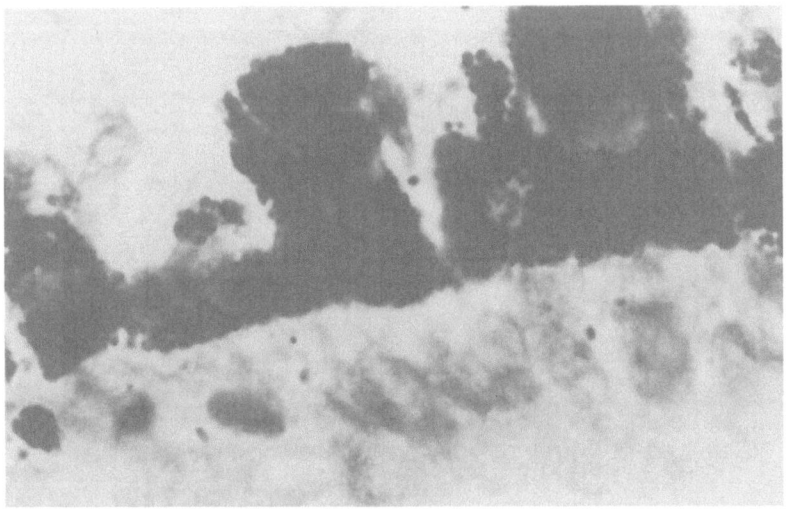

FIGURE 10. Microscopic appearance of the pigmented lesion located at the superior equator of OS. Note hyperplastic pigment epithelium. (H & E x960)

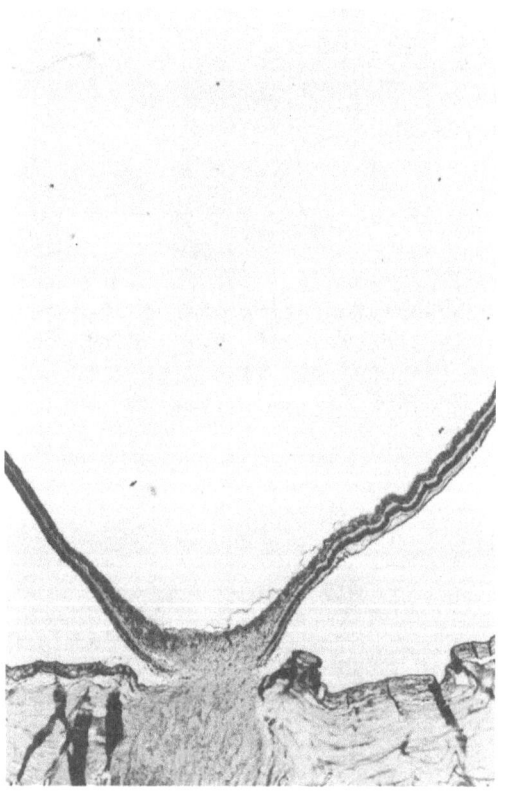

FIGURE 11.   Optic atrophy O.S.   (H & E x2.8)

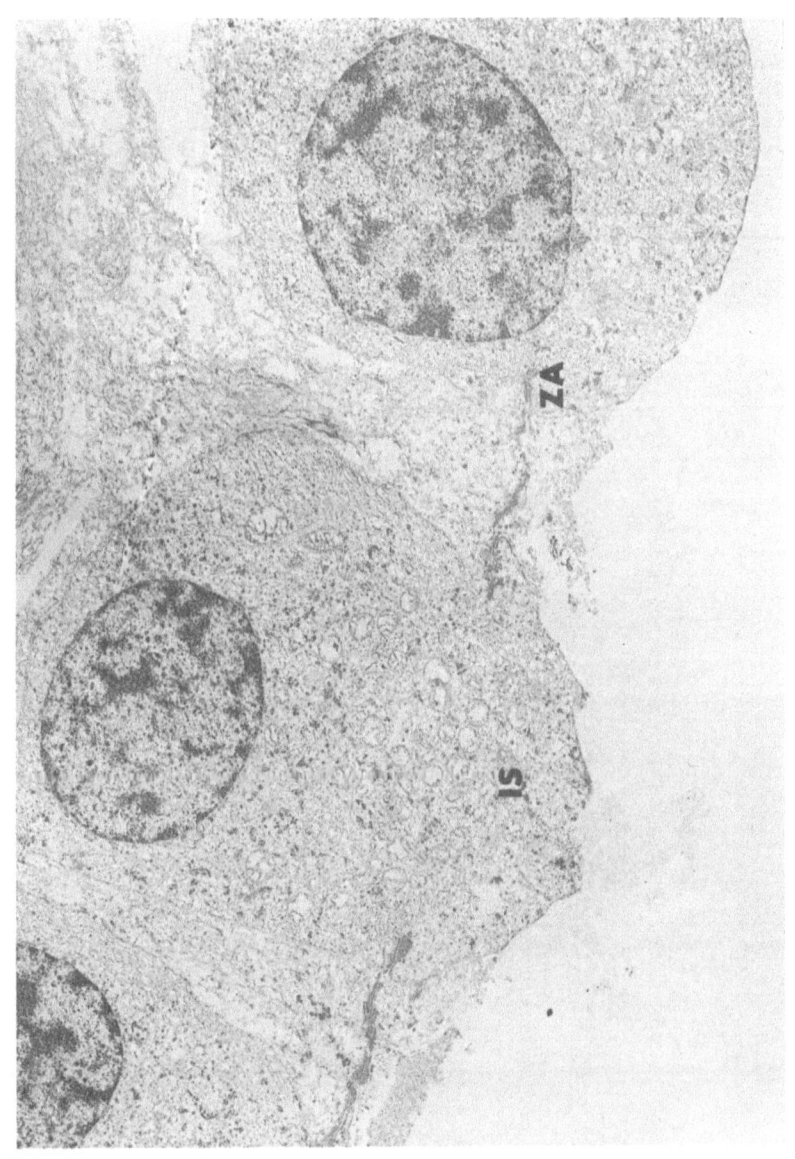

FIGURE 12. Electron micrograph of the outer nuclear monolayer in the left eye. Plump cone-like cells are present with the inner photoreceptor segments (IS) seen beyond the zonulae adherens of the external limiting membrane (ZA). Outer segments cannot be identified. (x6700)

DISCUSSION

Since the last half of the nineteenth century, there have been sporadic reports of pigmentary retinopathy occurring with polydactyly and other systemic abnormalities. In 1920, Bardet described a clinical entity comprised of pigmentary retinopathy associated with polydactyly, obesity, and genital hypoplasia. Two years later, Biedl added mental disability to this complex (Biedl, 1922), and this disorder was linked (Solis-Cohen and Weiss, 1925) to the cases described by Laurence and Moon in 1866. Franceschetti, Francois, and Babel (1963) and Botermans (1972) have reviewed this subject in considerable detail.

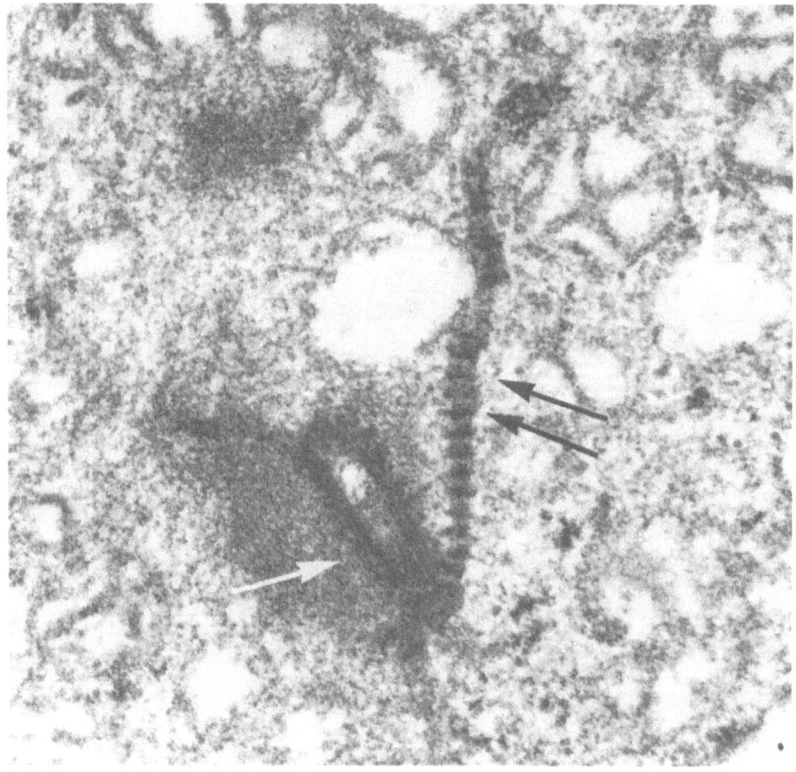

FIGURE 13. Basal body (arrow) and root filaments (two arrows) found in the remnant of an inner segment in the macular area. (x49,000)

A variety of types of pigmentary degenerations have been
described in this entity ranging from changes apparently clinically
indistinguishable from retinitis pigmentosa to salt and pepper type
chorioretinopathies, diffuse pigmentation of the posterior pole,
fundus albipunctatus, and retinitis pigmentosa sine pigmento. Few
of these cases, however, are documented with fundus photographs or
other illustrations. Most of the reports preceded the introduction
of the electroretinogram. In addition, there have been few histological reports documenting the microscopic changes seen in these
eyes. Rathmell and Burns (1938) implicated changes in the cerebral
cortex and brain stem suggestive of extensive embryonal dysplasia
as the cause for the visual disturbance. Brattgard, in 1949,
described fibrosis of the vascular layers of the capillary walls,

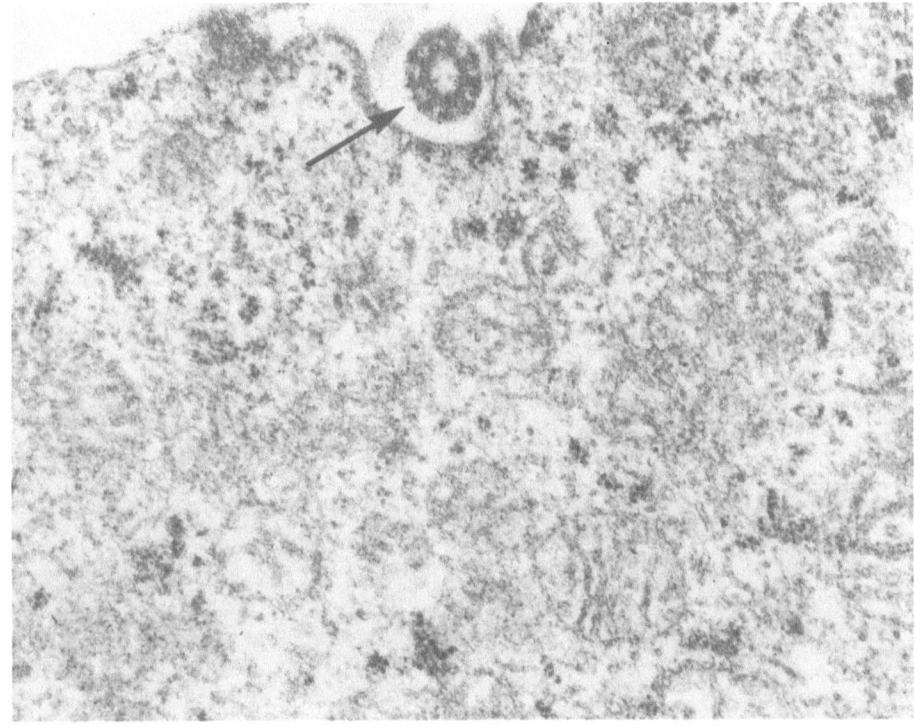

FIGURE 14. Cross section of a connecting cilium (arrow) found next
to a rudimentary inner segment. (x49,000)

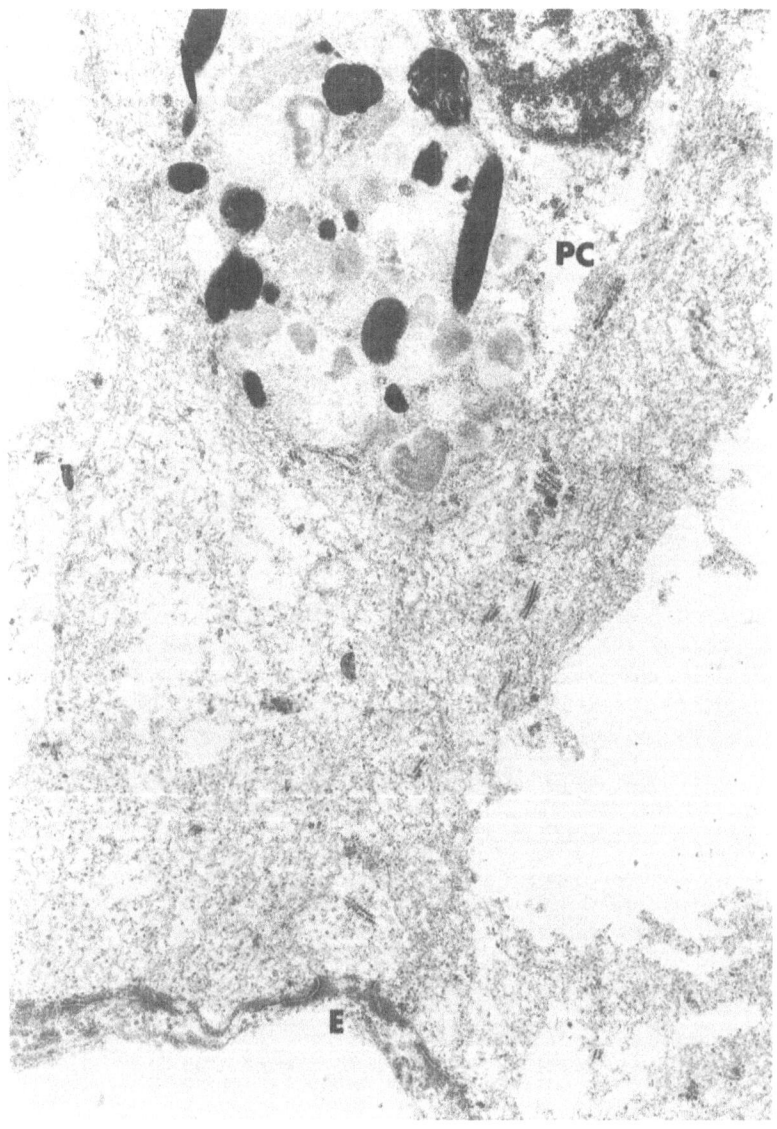

FIGURE 15.   Pigment laden cell within the retina. Pigmented cell
     (PC); external limiting membrane (E).   (x14,000)

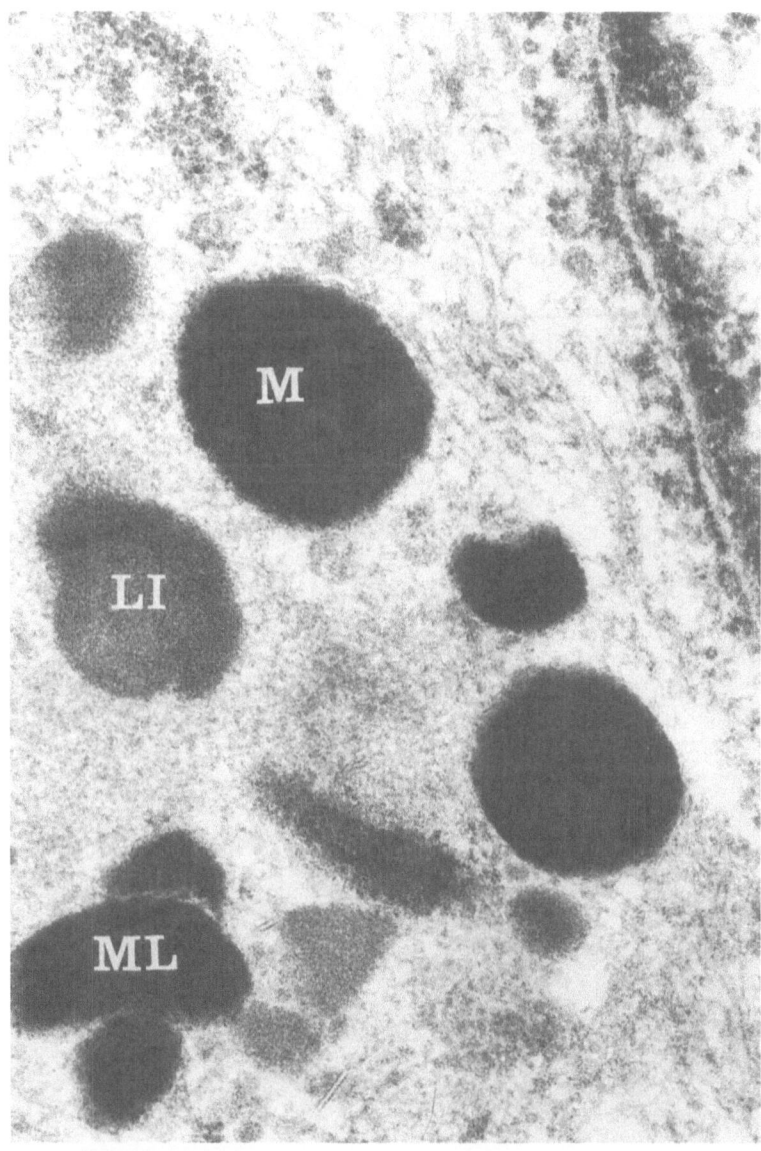

FIGURE 16. Higher magnification of the intraretinal pigment laden cell. Melanin (M), compound melanin-lipofuscin (ML), and lipid granules (LI) of variable size and granular density are seen. (x35,000)

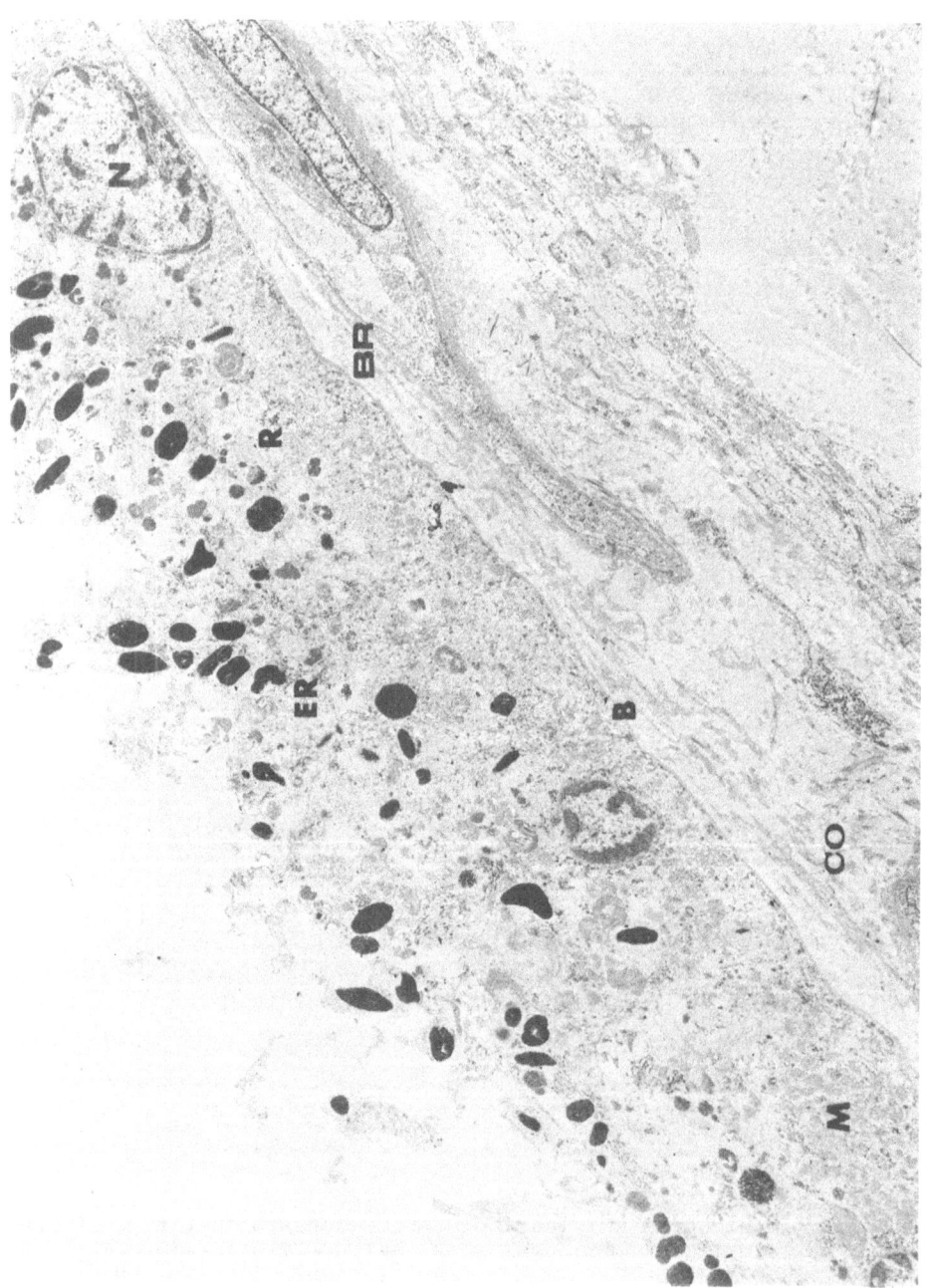

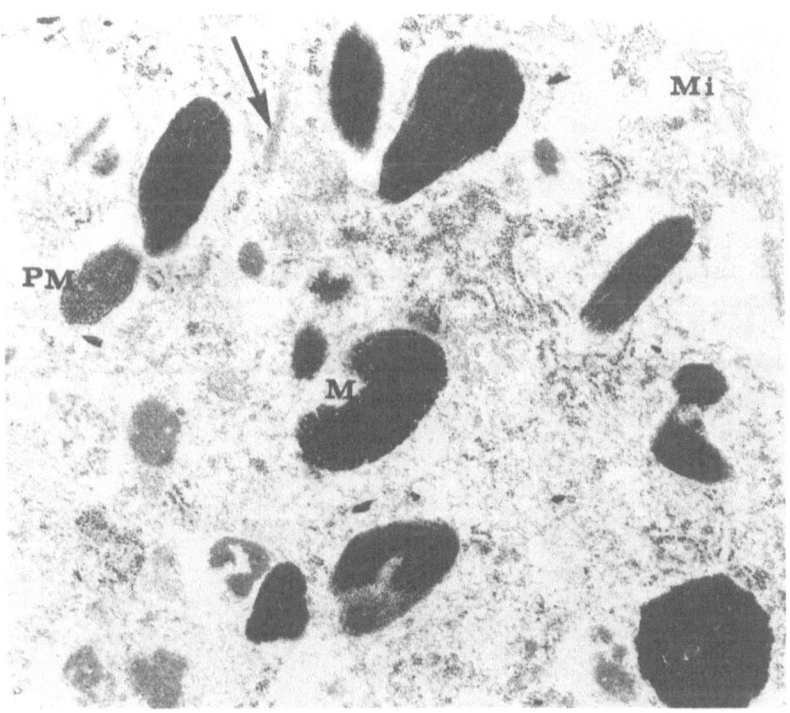

FIGURE 18. Higher magnification of a portion of the pigment epithelium illustrated in Fig. 15. Pigment granules (PM), melanin (M), rudiments of microville (Mi) and a cilium (arrow) are seen. (x14,000)

FIGURE 17. (facing page) Electron micrograph of the RPE showing pigment granules throughout the cytoplasm, but mostly confined to the apical portion of the cell. The nucleus (N) is located at the base of the cell; endoplasmic reticulum (ER), free ribosome (R), groups of mitochondria (M), and the basement membrane (B) are seen. (x5200)

a reduction in the number of photoreceptors in the retina, with
areas of complete disappearance of the outer nuclear layer and the
remaining cells in direct contact with Bruch's membrane. There
was loss of cells as well in the inner nuclear and ganglion cell
layers. Accumulation of pigment was seen about the fibrotic retinal vessels. A notable feature was the absence of abnormal changes
in the pigment epithelium.

    Bisland, in 1951, described a similar picture in a single eye
studied histopathologically from a 48 year old patient with LMBBS.
The changes were generally similar to those described by Brattgard
except for the presence of areas of total destruction of the pigment epithelium and photoreceptor cells.

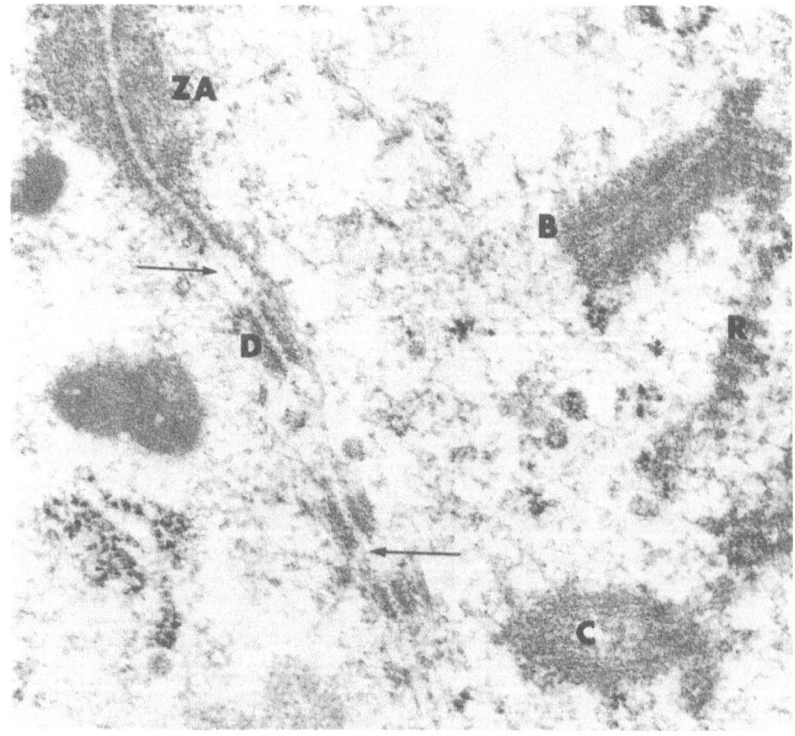

FIGURE 19. RPE showing the intercellular spaces (arrows), zonula
      adherens (ZA), and desmosomes (D). Basal body (B), rootlets
      (R), and a centriole (C) are also seen. (x49,000)

In an additional case described by Babel (1963) and subsequently by Franceschetti *et al.* (1963) and Ammann (1970), the diagnosis was less clear-cut and the case was interpreted to be an incomplete LMBBS. There was almost total destruction of the photoreceptor layer.

No electron microscopic descriptions of the retinal changes of LMBBS were found in the literature. It is apparent that the retinal changes may be variable and the relationship to other types of retinitis pigmentosa is not clear.

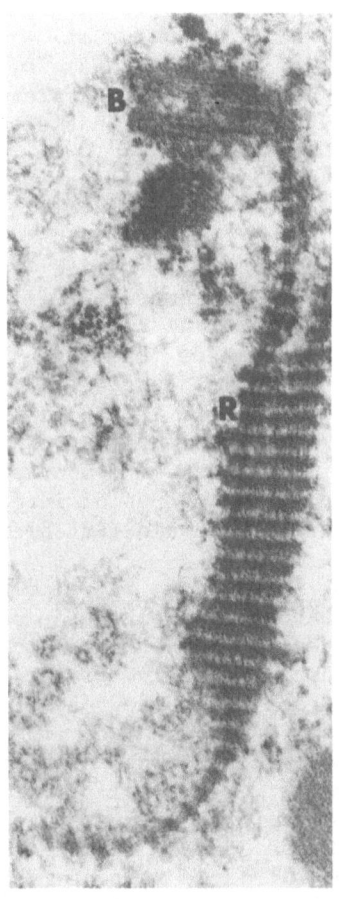

FIGURE 20. EM picture of a well-formed cross-striated rootlet (R) attached to a basal body (B) found in the RPE. (x72,000)

There have been only two reports of electron microscopic studies of the retina in various forms of human retinitis pigmentosa. Mizuno and Nishida (1967) described the changes in the eyes of two subjects who appeared to have an autosomally recessive form of the disease. They found remnants of cones at the posterior pole but none more anteriorly. There was "deterioration of the RPE membranes" in the area of visual cell loss with extension of RPE processes into the gaps between the photoreceptors. The retinal capillaries were hypocellular. Kolb and Gouras (1974) described the findings in the eyes of a 68 year old female with autosomally dominant retinitis pigmentosa. The only photoreceptors observed were foveal cones. The foveal RPE was found on electron microscopy to contain excessive amounts of lipofuscin in large spherical clusters and reduced amounts of melanin. The cells were positioned in different stages of migration away from Bruch's membrane. The large quantities of lipofuscin were interpreted as indicating the phagocytosis of outer segment material. In nonfoveal retinal patches the RPE contained little lipofuscin, but large amounts of melanin. These latter cells were interpreted as contributing to the "bone corpuscle" pigmentation in this disease.

The findings that the granules in the RPE and the intraretinal pigment-containing cells stained positively with oil red-0 indicate that these are true lipids (Lillie, 1954). The fact that the sudanophilia of the granules persisted in sections processed through the usual fat solvents needed for light microscopy preparation indicates that this material belongs to a lipid group which contains unsaturated fatty acids combined with proteins (Pearse, 1960). There was a relatively decreased lipofuscin stain in the RPE and only few granules in the intraretinal pigment laden cells gave a strong reaction to the lipofuscin stain (Luna, 1968). The positivity for the PAS stain, and the nonreactivity with acid fast stain places these lipids in a group of intermediate forms between "early" lipids and mature lipofuscin (Strehler, 1964).

In contrast to our LMBBS case, the pigment granules in the RPE of the retinitis pigmentosa patient were positive to lipofuscin stain and acid fast stain, and stained poorly with PAS, which places them in the mature lipofuscin group (Strehler, 1964). The intraretinal pigmented cells in the retinitis pigmentosa eye were completely negative for PAS stain and showed little evidence of lipofuscin. Abundant silver reducing substances were present which may indicate the presence of melanin (Pearse, 1960). Different staining characteristics of the pigmented cells over the malignant melanoma were noted. These showed marked staining with lipofuscin stain, slight staining with acid fast stain and strong reaction to PAS stain, which indicates a combination group of early and mature lipofuscin (Font, 1974).

The "normal" control eyes of the 4 year old possessed minimal amounts of sudanophilic granules, as would be expected (Streeten, 1961).

Electron microscopic examination of the cuboidal cells in the macular area of the left eye revealed rudimentary photoreceptor cells with no outer segments. In view of the almost total absence of photoreceptor outer segments in this young individual, the decreased stain for lipofuscin in the RPE can be explained by reduction in the amount of lipid available for ingestion by the pigment epithelium (Hogan, 1972).

The clinical history would indicate that the morphologic changes described above are in large part the result of degeneration rather than congenital hypoplasia, since the patient had 20/40 vision in both eyes (although with constricted fields and color blindness) when first seen. A progressive deterioration of visual function was subsequently documented.

ACKNOWLEDGEMENTS

This work was supported by USPHS Grant EY 00785-04.

REFERENCES

Ammann, F. (1970) Investigations cliniques et genetiques sur le syndrome de Bardet-Biedl en Suisse. *J. Genet. hum.* 18.

Babel, J. (1963) Constatations histologiques dans l'amaurose infantile de Leber et dans diverses formes d'hemeralopie. *Ophthalmologica (Basel)* 145:399-402.

Bardet, G. (1920) Sur un syndrome d'obesite infantile avec polydactylie et retinite pigmentaire. (Contributions a l'etude des formes cliniques et o'obesite hypophysaire.) Thesis, Paris.

Biedl, A. (1922) Ein Geschwisterpaar mit adiposogenitaler Dystrophie. *Dtsch. med. Wschr.* 48:1630.

Bisland, T. (1951) The Laurence-Moon-Biedl syndrome. Report of a typical case with complete necropsy. *Amer. J. Ophthal.* 34: 874-885.

Botermans, C. H. (1972) Primary pigmentary retinal degeneration and its association with neurological diseases, in "Handbook of Clinical Neurology" (P. J. Vinken and G. W. Bruyn, eds.) p. 148, American Elsevier, New York.

Brattgard, S. O. (1949) The pathology of Laurence-Moon-Biedl syndrome. *Acta path. microbiol. scand.* 26:525-538.

Font, R. L., Zimmerman, L. E., and Armaly, M. F. (1974) The nature of the orange pigment over a choroidal melanoma. *Arch. Ophthal.* 91:359-362.

Franceschetti, A., Francois, J., and Babel, J. (1963) "Les heredo-degenerescences, chorioretiniennes. (Degenerescences tapeto-retiniennes," Vols. I en II, Masson, Paris.

Hogan, M. J. (1972) Role of the retinal pigment epithelium in macular diseases. *Trans. Amer. Acad. Ophthal. Otolaryngol.* 76:64-80.

Kolb, H., and Gouras, P. (1974) Electron microscopic observations of human retinitis pigmentosa. *Invest. Ophthal.* 13:487-498.

Laurence, J. Z., and Moon, R. C. (1866) Four cases of retinitis pigmentosa occurring in the same family and accompanied by general imperfections of development. *Ophthal. Rev.* (old series) 2:32-41.

Lillie, R. D. (1954) "Histopathologic Technique and Practical Histochemistry," The Blakiston Division, McGraw-Hill, New York.

Luna, L. G. (ed.) (1968) "Manual of Histologic Staining, Methods of the Armed Forces Institute of Pathology," ed. 3, p. 186, The Blakiston Division, McGraw-Hill, New York.

Mizuno, K., and Nishida, S. (1967) Electron microscopic studies of human retinitis pigmentosa. *Amer. J. Ophthal.* 63:791-803.

Pearse, A. G. E. (1960). "Histochemistry, Theoretical and Applied," Little, Brown and Company, Boston.

Rathmell, T. K., and Burns, M. A. (1938) The Laurence-Biedl syndrome occurring in a brother and sister. *Arch. Neurol. Psychiat.* 39:1033-1042.

Solis-Cohen, S., and Weiss, E. (1925) Dystrophia adiposogenitalis with atypical retinitis pigmentosa and mental deficiency (Laurence-Biedl syndrome). *Amer. J. Med. Sci.* 169:489-505.

Streeten, B. W. (1961) The sudanophilic granules of the human retinal pigment epithelium. *Arch. Ophthal.* 66:391-398.

Strehler, B. L. (1964) On the histochemistry and ultrastructure of age pigment. *Adv. Gerontol. Res.* 1:343-384.

Tso, M. O. M., Fine, B. S., and Zimmerman, L. E. (1970) The nature
of retinoblastoma. II. Photoreceptor differentiation, an
electron microscopy study. *Amer. J. Ophthal.* 69:350-359.

DISCUSSION OF THE PAPER

DR. BERGSMA: I have a comment, and that is that most of the
reports in the literature on Laurence-Moon-Biedl talk about atypical retinitis pigmentosa and the few that have been well studied
I think fall into the category of cone-rod degeneration.

DR. BUYUKMIHCI: Yes, that is true. We do not present this
case as a typical case of retinitis pigmentosa, but more as a finding of a retinitis pigmentosa-like syndrome with an interesting
pathology.

DR. BERGSMA: In a case that has progressed this far, and with
the unreliability that some of these patients have, it is hard to
differentiate, but I think it is more likely that this is cone-rod
degeneration and not typical RP.

DR. BUYUKMIHCI: I agree. It is unfortunate that this patient
was not examined very early in life with more objective testing to
find out if there was a developmental abnormality.

DR. TSO: Did you have an opportunity to study the pigment
cells surrounding the blood vessels? If you did, what were the
pathologic characteristics?

DR. BUYUKMIHCI: I thought I presented one. One of the micro-
graphs was supposed to represent one of the pigment cells that had
migrated into the retina.

DR. TSO: Do they have epithelial characteristics, or are they
phagocytes?

DR. BUYUKMIHCI: They seem to have characteristics of both
epithelium and phagocytes. We couldn't be sure what they were.

DR. DOWLING: In normal pigment epithelial cells you occasionally will see a cilium with basal body and rootlet and that I think
you cannot relate to a disease process. It happens occasionally.

DR. BUYUKMIHCI: We weren't sure whether this was a response
of degeneration or whether it was just a more unusual finding of a
normal thing. But we found it often in this eye in comparison to
other eyes.

DR. LAVAIL: Were there any regions where all of the photoreceptors were missing--any patches?

DR. BUYUKMIHCI: Oh, yes. In the macular area there were no
photoreceptor cells *per se*--I mean, there were nuclei and inner
segments, but there was no outer segment material at all and there
appeared to be no phagosomes in the retinal pigment epithelium.
But there were outer segments present peripherally, which probably
accounted for the little vision that the patient had.

DR. WOLBARSHT: We found an old German paper describing the
pathology of an intermediate case and we were hoping to drag it in
and hit you over the head with it, but unfortunately all they
described was what they called a fatty degeneration. It was un-
clear, first, that the patient had retinitis pigmentosa and second,
what they meant by "fatty degeneration." I was hoping, of course,
that it said lipid-like rod debris, but that unfortunately was not
the case.

DR. BUYUKMIHCI: Well, we have a lot of lipofuscin-like
material in this case. I don't know if that corresponds with fatty
degeneration or not.

DR. WOLBARSHT: I don't know either. There were no pictures.

RESEARCH MODELS FOR RETINITIS PIGMENTOSA

INTRODUCTION

John E. Dowling

The Biological Laboratories
Harvard University
Cambridge, Massachusetts   02138

Among investigators who are studying retinitis pigmentosa there is a genuine optimism that in the not-too-distant future, we will begin to understand the underlying causes of this tragic disease. One of the main reasons for this optimism is that we have available today a number of animal models with genetically-linked retinal diseases that resemble retinitis pigmentosa and similar degenerative lesions. Having such laboratory animals with which to work, to study, and on which to test ideas is an advantage that cannot be overestimated. Some years ago, for example, it was observed that in rats suffering from retinal dystrophy, the progress of the disease could be slowed by maintaining the animals in dim illumination. As a result of this and other observations, several clinical programs are now under way to test if the progress of retinitis pigmentosa in the human can be slowed by restricting light to the eye (see Section III of this book).

So far there have been discovered genetically-linked retinal lesions that appear relevant to retinitis pigmentosa in that the photoreceptor cells appear to be primarily affect in mice, rats, and dogs, and I suspect that if we search further, we will find similar diseases in many more species. Photoreceptor cells in vertebrates appear to be particularly susceptible to degenerative lesions, for reasons that are not yet clear. The recent discovery that vertebrate receptor cells appear to be *on* all the time in the dark and that light turns them *off* indicates they are a most unusual cell metabolically and perhaps provides us with an important clue.

Mice with an inherited retinal degenerative disease were first described and studied with a variety of techniques by Clyde Keeler working at the Massachusetts Eye and Ear Infirmary in Boston in the 1920's. Keeler appeared to be far ahead of his time, for no one continued work with these animals until field mice with retinal degeneration were discovered in Switzerland in the 1950's.

Rats with a retinitis pigmentosa-like degeneration were discovered in England in the late 1930's, carefully maintained through the war outside London at Mill Hill, and brought to this country by Richard Sidman in 1960. Since then there has been active interest in these animals, and this interest is rapidly growing.

Reports of dogs with retinitis pigmentosa-like diseases date back to the beginning of this century, but today we still know very little about the canine retinal lesions, far less, for example, than we know about the diseases in the mouse and rat. There may be as many as five different retinal degenerative diseases in the dog, all of which will be of great interest and importance to study in depth.

The following presentations provide a flavor of the type of research that has been and can be carried out on the research models for retinitis pigmentosa. As noted above, much of the attention on animal models for the past 15 years has been focused on the rat with retinal dystrophy, and several of the contributions of this section reflect the emphasis on this model. But as is also noted above, the canine models may be of enormous value and as yet we know too little about them. I think we can look forward with confidence to continued and probably to accelerated progress in our use of animal models for an understanding of retinitis pigmentosa and related retinal degenerations.

SOME ANIMAL MODELS OF RETINITIS PIGMENTOSA

Werner K. Noell

Neurosensory Laboratory
University of Buffalo
Buffalo, New York

(Summary by M. L. Wolbarsht from conference recording)

The relevance of the animal models discussed in this symposium
to the human disease is at best a very tentative one, even though
several excellent presentations have been made on the physiological
and pathological properties of photoreceptors and pigment epithelium in various animals, which seem to deserve consideration in
such a comparison. The specific models for retinitis pigmentosa
include hereditary anomalies which differ with species along the
vertebrate and even invertebrate scale, as well as the effects of
chemical and physical agents.

It is appropriate to start this review with some reference to
some earlier work of my own. In the rhesus monkey iodoacetic acid
appears to produce a pathology similar to retinitis pigmentosa.
It kills almost all of the rods but does not touch the cones. In
the parafoveal region cones survive, but they undergo drastic
changes when they spread into the missing spaces, due to the death
of the rods. Further away from the fovea, in the far periphery,
we see what looks like a typical picture of retinitis pigmentosa.
Only the cone nuclei are left with the pigment epithelium moved
toward the inner surface of the retina. In some places the retina
is pigmented and others not, while many of the nuclei have migrated
in from the pigment epithelium. Iodoacetic acid appears, partially
at least, to inhibit glycolosis, and in this case the rods and
cones differ greatly in their survival when the ordinary metabolic
activity is impaired. The iodoacetate effect, with some differences, is present in all mammals. In the rabbit the iodoacetate
appears to act first not on the inner or outer segment, but on the
synaptic terminals, showing that this is the most energy dependent
location in the cell. The b-wave drops out first, showing that
synaptic transmission between the rods and the next neuron is

inhibited earliest.   This effect can be shown not only by disturbance to the metabolism (and especially by the specific metabolism
producing APT through the glycolytic system) but also by x-irradiation, and in the rabbit by high oxygen tension.   The effect of
x-irradiation on high oxygen indicates that something more is
affected while just metabolism, possibly a membrane bound activity.
All changes occur very rapidly. A single typical dose of irradia-
tion of perhaps 20 or 30 minutes will make everything drop out,
such as normal oxygen consumption, electroretinogram, and ordinary
metabolism.   It seems to cause a change in some membranes which are
equally distributed in the cell, a change which can spread to other
cells immediately. The high oxygen effect in the rabbit is also
very interesting. The visual cells die within days when the rabbit
is left in an atmosphere of 70 to 80% oxygen.   The effect is similar to that of x-irradiation as the photoreceptors are initially
affected while the bipolar cells and ganglion cells are normal, and
the damage to the pigment epithelium seems minor.   From this it
appears that the visual cells are something very special.   This
oxygen effect may be limited to the rods as the rabbit has very few
cones in the part of the retina we have examined.

    The next topic to be covered is the genetic controlled defects
of the rat.   It is well that we are not rats with this particular
genetic defect, for even a little bit of light causes a marked
change in the eyes of these animals.   The visual cells, their
nuclei, the bipolar cells, and the Mueller cells--almost all disappear with just 24 hours of strong light (150 foot candles).
After the visual cells disappear the pigment epithelium also disappears.   The effect is an area one and is dependent upon the time
of exposure to light.   Twelve hours causes less, 48 hours more,
by increasing the area of the retina in which the visual cells
have died.   Continued light exposure causes an increasing scotoma.
The size of this scotoma can be quantified by the progressive
disappearance of the electroretinogram from the still somewhat
functional remaining area of the retina.   It seems certain that
the light acts directly on the rhodopsin, that is, the effect is
initiated by the action of light on the rhodopsin.   There is
massive visual cell death if 90% of the rhodopsin is kept bleached
for one or two days.

    The real question is, how can light do this?   In these rats
the damage by light is unbelievably dependent on temperature.   A
small rise in body temperature to 100° to 102°F enhances the effect
manyfold.   It brings on the peak effect faster and emphasizes the
difference between continuous and cyclic light exposures. If an
animal has been kept for a week in complete darkness, a strong
light is much more dangerous than if an animal has been kept in a
weak, cyclic light--12 hours on, 12 hours off.

The rat is an exceptional animal with respect to response to damage by light. Other nocturnal animals, including the nocturnal moth, are also damaged by light, but they require much higher light intensity and a longer exposure time. What happens in this rat is something special, probably due to the genetic makeup of the photoreceptors in the rat making them more susceptible to light. Rats kept from the age of 21 days to 56 days in cyclic light, 12 hours on and 12 hours off at 5 foot candles intensity (too low for us to read with), were compared with another group kept in complete darkness. Both groups were exposed to 100 foot candles of green light. The animals kept in the dark lost 90% of the a-wave. The group raised in cyclic light were exposed to the same green light for exactly the same time and the changes in the eye were very small, very slight. If the rats raised in the dark were put into cyclic light, and those raised in cyclic light put into darkness, each gradually assumes the susceptibilities of the other. Darkness and light are not exactly interchangeable, but depend upon the past history of the animal.

We have recently attempted to measure some of the changes in the animals which have been kept in darkness versus light, and we see a difference in rhodopsin. In light the rhodopsin concentration is lower. Also, the phospholipid/rhodopsin ratio is much higher in the cyclic light group than in the dark, which indicates that the phospholipid protein in the photoreceptors differs between the groups. There is also a difference in the highly unsaturated fatty acids characteristic of the outer segment and synaptic membranes. In this case the fatty acid phosphatidylethanolamine is almost half unsaturated. It is possible that these highly unsaturated fatty acids make the system more susceptible to oxidation, especially auto-oxidation. Perhaps also light has, in this system, the pathological capacity to cause oxidation of membrane constituents or perhaps auto-oxidation is coupled with the renewal mechanism for the discs. As Richard Young mentioned earlier in the symposium, the pigment epithelium apparently remains intact when visual cells die, although there is an accumulation of rhodopsin debris between the retina and pigment epithelium. An animal kept in the dark for 83 days loses its visual cells and rod outer segment debris accumulates. This debris has a different phospholipid and a different fatty acid concentration as compared with the normal outer segment. In the rat the debris is 80 to 90% outer segments, which seem to accumulate because of a lack of phagocytic function in the pigment epithelium and this debris is the cause of the pigment epithelium degeneration. A dystrophic rat kept in the dark from birth to 27 days has a normal retina, while a litter mate of the same age, after exposure for 24 hours to 150 foot candles, has light damage. The pigment epithelium disappears due to the effect of light along with most of the photoreceptors. There are no inner and outer segments and relatively few nuclei. As John Dowling first pointed out, the susceptibility of these young rats to damage by light is remarkably high. Cyclic light at 5 foot candles protects normal rats against light damage, but the hereditarily dystrophic rats must be bred in total darkness. Cyclic light does not protect them. On the contrary, weak cyclic light, as low as 2 (or even 1) foot candles, destroys the visual cells. After three days the electroretinogram is depressed. Longer exposures or older animals give even more marked effects.

My current hypothesis is that the bleaching of rhodopsin, in the rat at least, decreases the structural chemical stability of the rod outer segment membrane. Non-bleached rhodopsin, probably by protein lipid interaction, provides the membrane with a particular stability which makes it resistant to the damaging effects of light. We find that the damaging effect of light originates in the rhodopsin in the outer segment. The normal rat only shows this effect when the rhodopsin is bleached, but the dystrophic rat has this abnormal membrane structure even without exposure to light. This, I feel, is a chemical reaction--similar to the effects from x-rays, high oxygen, or exposure to light. All of those indicate that lipid peroxidation is the cause of cell death. It is still a mystery how an effect initiated in the outer segments by light affects the pigment epithelium. Perhaps strong outer segment damage has a toxic effect which spreads to the pigment epithelium.

Perhaps from all this may come some ideas for the management of the human disease. The relevance, of course, depends upon the similarity, and we have yet to prove a similarity between the human disease and the animal disease. In 1969 we examined the retinal capillary network by Kuwabara's technique. The capillaries are isolated by trypsin digestion. The vasoconstriction or abnormality of degeneration appeared in the hereditary dystrophic rat after the debris accumulated and the outer nuclear layer disappeared. However, in human retinitis pigmentosa, vasoconstriction is an early phenomenon. We do not know of any debris, so we must assume that there is a change in the oxygen distribution within the retina. This is an important point. However, the response of the vascular system may be an indication of debris accumulation in humans.

DISCUSSION OF THE PAPER

DR. MEHAFFEY: Dr. Noell, does the degeneration of the RCS rat proceed in total darkness?

DR. NOELL: Oh, yes.

DR. MEHAFFEY: It seems that you are proposing that light is what triggers off the degeneration.

DR. NOELL: Oh, no. It triggers it off in the normal rat. The hereditary rat has a membrane abnormality to a different degree --qualitatively, quantitatively different degree--than the normal rat, plus other things. There is also a pigment epithelial abnormality. Nobody who has made any proposal has, over the last 10-20 years, considered what kind of gene action is involved. Is a structural gene involved? From my own work on the heredity of the mouse I am very certain that it isn't a structural gene, but is one of those so-called regulatory genes--regulatory or processing genes, and this action is much more difficult to get a handle on than at the structural gene. You have to link some degenerative activity to particular genetic tests and this can prove your point. This is the answer to that problem.

DR. HERRON. Dr. Noell, you stated that you were certain that the rod outer segment production removal defect in the RCS rat was not the cause of the subsequent photoreceptor cell death. The rat shows a decreased renewal rate of rod outer segment material as time goes on. Regular photoreceptor outer segment production seems to follow quite rapidly when you are looking at them under phase scope examination, so obviously these normal outer segments fall apart in a not-normal environment. And then if the photoreceptor area is felt to be fed nutritionally from the choriocapillaris, then could not the debris accumulation be significant in creating a barrier here?

DR. NOELL: I can give you no hard facts about what I said. It is a hypothesis, of course. I said, "I am sure." That doesn't mean it is the truth. This is a theory that the diffusion of oxygen and nutrients is impaired to the extent that the retina dies-- the photoreceptors die. The photoreceptors, especially with regard to oxygen, are very, very resistant to a metabolic change. My best argument against this is (1) that the light destroys--light destroys in no time, and accelerates the existing tendency, so to speak--even this very, very weak light. Light, so far as we know, does not increase oxygen consumption; on the contrary, it reduces oxygen consumption of the photoreceptors. Another reason is that if you separate the retina, and I have separated many retinas from the pigment epithelium--with big distances in between. It is very, very unusual to find the loss of outer nuclei. This is pathological visual cell death as manifested by the disappearance of outer nuclei. Whatever causes a detachment is followed by this with much delay. What gets destroyed quickly is the outer segment with the inner segment, but the nucleus is very, very resistant.

VISUAL CELL RENEWAL SYSTEMS AND THE PROBLEM OF RETINITIS PIGMENTOSA

Richard W. Young

Department of Anatomy and Jules Stein Eye Institute
UCLA School of Medicine
Los Angeles, California 90024

INTRODUCTION

The recent growth of our understanding of renewal systems in rods and cones has opened up new ways of thinking about the visual cells. We are beginning to realize that the apparently imperturbable structure of these long-lived cells is actually in continual flux. Their basic constituents--the molecules, membranes and organelles of which they are composed--are in a perpetual state of dynamic renovation, due to extremely complex mechanisms of balanced degradation and reassembly. These renewal systems are as much a part of their inherent nature as is the ability to convert the absorption of light into a visual message.

The gradual deepening of our awareness of these exquisitely regulated processes allows us to look beyond questions of how they normally protect the rods and cones from the ravages of injury and aging, and to ask what might result if these renewal pathways were disturbed through genetic defect or disease. When we examine the problem of retinitis pigmentosa from this point of view, it seems likely that one or more of the several forms of this disease may result from a derangement of renewal pathways, and, further, that the differential effects on rods and cones in retinitis pigmentosa and related genetic diseases may arise from intrinsic differences in the renewal mechanisms of the two classes of visual cells.

RETINITIS PIGMENTOSA

Retinitis pigmentosa (RP) is one of the most common of all the inherited eye disorders. The age of onset of symptoms varies considerably. Night blindness, the earliest symptom, may appear in childhood, or later, but almost always it begins before the age of 30. Thereafter, it is slowly progressive in both eyes. The visual field gradually contracts from the periphery, so that central vision persists the longest. Jet-black, spidery spots of pigment are the earliest ophthalmoscopic signs, but these are secondary effects, and may not develop until years after the first symptoms. They occur most commonly in the equatorial region, generally near the vessels, and in the approximate zone where the first field defect is observed. This abnormal pigmentation tends to spread as the disease progresses. In advanced stages, the retinal blood vessels are narrowed, and the choroidal circulation may come into view due to pigment epithelium migration and atrophy (Roberts, 1970; Sorsby, 1972).

Retinitis pigmentosa shows considerable variation in degree, age of onset of symptoms, course, prognosis, and inheritance, due to the fact that it can be caused by the action of several different abnormal genes.

The most common mode of transmission is autosomal recessive (Francois, 1961; Jay, 1972). It is very likely that several recessive genes are involved (Roberts, 1970; Sorsby, 1972). There is also an autosomal dominant form, which usually develops later and is less severe (Francois, 1961). The majority of families with dominantly inherited RP have shown complete penetrance. Skipping of one or two generations has been described in a few families, however. This implies the existence of a dominant form with reduced penetrance (Berson *et al.*, 1969b). The sex-linked form is the least common, but the most severe, producing a rapid progression in the affected male, often leading to blindness by the age of 20 (Sorsby, 1972; Jay, 1972; Jay and Bird, 1973). Some authors have suggested that the sex-linked form should be subdivided into recessive, dominant, and intermediate types, because of the great variability in the carrier females (Roberts, 1970; Sorsby, 1972).

The presence of additional defective genes which may provoke retinitis pigmentosa is shown by the existence of several hereditary syndromes in which retinitis pigmentosa represents only one of multiple components. Among these are Usher's syndrome (Cherry, 1972), Alström's syndrome (Alström *et al.*, 1959), Cockayne's syndrome (Cockayne, 1936), Laurence-Moon-Bardet-Biedl syndrome (Francois, 1969), Refsum's syndrome, Bassen-Kornzweig syndrome, and amaurotic familial idiocy (a group of disorders including gangliosidoses and lipidoses) (Francois, 1975), as well as several mucopolysaccharidoses: Hurler's disease (MPS I), Hunter's disease (MPS II), Sanfillipo's disease (MPS III), and Scheie's disease (MPS V) (Francois, 1974b). All of these show autosomal recessive inheritance, except for Hunter's disease, which is sex-linked recessive.

Hereditary disorders are caused by defects in the genetic code which result in abnormal animal acid composition in specific pro- teins.   If the affected protein is coded by a gene which is activated in only one type of cell,   then the primary effect will be localized in that cell,   perhaps even totally restricted to it-- although a primary lesion in one cell type often leads to secondary effects in other cells. For example, the effects of defective cod- ing for a visual pigment protein will be restricted to one type of visual cell without direct effects on other types of cells.   In contrast, a defective protein which is required as an enzyme by many different types of cells throughout the body will clearly have widespread primary effects, and probably secondary effects as well.

Consequently, retinitis pigmentosa unaccompanied by extraocular lesions is probably due to defective genes which are activated only in the retina, whereas retinitis pigmentosa which occurs as a compo- nent of a complex syndrome with accompanying effects outside the eye is evidently the result of abnormal genes activated in other types of cells, possibly including retinal cells as well.

The few available histopathological reports describing retinas with RP unfortunately all deal with the late stages of degeneration, often 20 or more years after total or near total blindness, and fre- quently with less than optimal tissue preservation.   Significantly, the final appearance is remarkably similar, no matter what the gene- tic form of the disease (Gonin, 1903; Leber, 1915; Verhoeff, 1931; Cogan, 1950; Lucas, 1956; Wolter, 1957; Mizuno and Nishida, 1967; Kolb and Gouras, 1974). The primary abnormality is the disappear- ance of the rods and cones. (A few abnormally short and thick cones may survive in the central area.) The inner retinal layers appear relatively normal, except for some gliosis, and variable amounts of pigment invasion, particularly along blood vessels.   There may be depigmentation, thinning, degeneration or proliferation of the pig- ment epithelium.   These changes are usually most pronounced in the periphery.

Gonin (1903) thought that a slight atrophy of the choriocapil- laris might be the cause of the rod and cone degeneration, but this idea has had little support. Most studies indicate that the chorio- capillaris is not affected (Leber, 1915; Verhoeff, 1931; Cogan, 1950; Carr, 1972; Archer *et al.*, 1972).

Leber (1915), Cogan (1950) and others were convinced that the primary lesion is in the visual cells.   Recent electrophysiological studies of individuals with RP have strengthened this conclusion-- although they do not exclude the possibility that the defect may reside in the pigment epithelium, which is known to be intimately involved in the metabolic activities of the rods and cones. Delays in rod ERG implicit times have been demonstrated in the early stages of all the progressive forms of retinitis pigmentosa (Berson, 1975,

1976). This delay is believed to indicate that there is widespread
involvement of all or nearly all of the rods across the retina.
[Cone responses are also delayed in implicit time in dominant RP
with reduced penetrance (Berson *et al.*, 1969b), autosomal recessive
retinitis pigmentosa (Berson, 1976), and sex-linked retinitis
pigmentosa (Berson *et al.*, 1969a).   In contrast, patients with
localized retinal disease, such as dominant sector retinitis pigmentosa, have normal rod and cone ERG implicit times (Berson and
Howard, 1971; Berson, 1975).] Furthermore, the amplitude of the
early receptor potential is reduced well below normal in all
patients who have been tested (Berson and Goldstein, 1970a, 1970b).
Changes in the early receptor potential indicate that the visual
cell outer segments are affected.

     In summary, there are several distinct diseases grouped under
the heading "retinitis pigmentosa." Each is caused by a different
defective gene. Some of these abnormal genes are activated only in
the retina; some are activated in cells located in other parts of
the body as well. In every case, however, the predominant effect
in the eye is the gradual degeneration of the visual cells.

                    PROGRESSIVE CONE DEGENERATIONS

     In retinitis pigmentosa, the symptoms and ERG analyses indi-
cate that the rods are usually affected most severely, although
cones may show functional abnormalities upon electrophysiological
testing very early in the disease (Berson *et al.*, 1969a, 1969b;
Berson and Goldstein, 1970b; Berson, 1976). In recent years, it
has become evident that there are also a number of inherited retinal degenerations which primarily affect cones (Sloan and Brown,
1962).

     Many authors subdivide these disorders into "progressive cone
degenerations," with little or no rod abnormality, and "progressive
cone-rod degenerations," where symptoms relating to the cone dysfunction predominate, but the rods are also affected (Goodman
et al., 1963; Berson *et al.*, 1968a, 1968b). The major symptoms are
loss of visual acuity, bilateral central scotomas, photophobia, and
defective color vision. Loss of peripheral vision and night blindness, classic RP symptoms, are extremely rare complaints (Krill
et al., 1973).   In all of these diseases, the time when symptoms
first appear is variable, but generally occurs in childhood, before
the age of 20. Autosomal recessive inheritance is recorded,
although autosomal dominant appears as a more common mode of transmission (Deutman, 1971; Krill *et al.*, 1973; Francois *et al.*, 1974;
Pearlman *et al.*, 1974).   The variable inheritance, variable severity and rate of progression indicate that several defective genes
are involved.

A related hereditary retinal degeneration is Stargardt's disease, which is autosomal recessive (Deutman, 1974; Francois, 1974a). In this condition, a central scotoma with abnormal color vision develops. The foveal cones are destroyed, and both rods and cones degenerate in the immediately surrounding area. The pigment epithelium also degenerates in this zone (Blodi, 1966). Among several additional inherited macular degenerations are pericentral retinitis pigmentosa, which is autosomal recessive, and vitelliform dystrophy, which is autosomal dominant (Deutman, 1974; Francois, 1974a).

DECREASED LONGEVITY OF VISUAL CELLS

For an extended period comprising many years after birth, individuals afflicted with these hereditary diseases are unaware of any visual deficit, may be completely free of any ophthalmological signs of abnormality, and show normal visual fields by conventional perimetric testing. Nevertheless, the defective gene is almost certainly operative throughout this entire period, having been activated prior to birth. It may be assumed that all of the genes which underlie the functional activities of fully developed cells are activated when those cells undergo differentiation. Renewal pathways which rejuvenate mature visual cells, for example, have been detected in operation before cell development is completed (Young, 1967; LaVail, 1973).

Sensitive electrophysiological tests have revealed abnormalities in rod and cone function (subnormal and delayed ERG) prior to the development of ophthalmological changes, in young siblings of individuals affected with dominant and recessive forms of RP (Berson, 1973, 1976). These abnormalities may represent a manifestation of the defective gene which precedes cellular degeneration.

Retinitis pigmentosa and the allied cone diseases arise from multiple genetic abnormalities, all of which provoke the degeneration of rods and cones. The similarity of the end state suggests that the hereditary defects may disturb different aspects of the same or closely related processes. The altered genes do not prevent the differentiation of the rods and cones, but they are incompatible with their long-term survival. Longevity of the visual cells is reduced. It therefore seems reasonable to suggest that the defective genes may disrupt processes which are essential for the maintenance of the mature cells--that is, renewal systems.

VISUAL CELL RENEWAL SYSTEMS

Although the concept that many of the body's constituents are in a "dynamic state" was expressed more than 30 years ago (Schoenheimer, 1942), the realization that the components of the visual cells also undergo turnover was not established until quite recently, when the technique of autoradiography was used to chart the fate within the retina of molecules labeled with radioisotopes (Nover and Schultze, 1960; Maraini and Franguelli, 1962; Maraini et al., 1963; Droz, 1963; Young, 1965-1967; Ocumpaugh and Young, 1966; Bok, 1966). Now the outlines of some of the major renewal pathways are beginning to come into focus. Each of these pathways involves multiple steps, requiring enzymes and other specific proteins (such as membrane receptors and carrier proteins). Some require participation by the pigment epithelium. All of them have to be integrated with one another. Thus, there are abundant opportunities for defects in the genetic code to disturb renewal mechanisms, gradually creating imbalances which eventually could lead to death.

There is direct evidence from autoradiographic experiments that all of the major classes of molecules--proteins, carbohydrates and lipids--are incessantly renewed in the visual cells and pigment epithelium. The only compound which appears to be stable is nuclear DNA--the genetic material itself (Schultze et al., 1961; Sidman, 1961).

The activated portions of the DNA, however, are continually engaged in the production of RNA molecules (Bok, 1970; Young and Bok, 1970; Koenig, 1971). Much, but not all, of the RNA is then transferred from the nucleus to the cytoplasm (specifically, the myoid zone in visual cells). The different species of RNA (messenger, transfer, and ribosomal) then mediate the assembly of amino acids into specific proteins. In the visual cells (Young, 1967; Young and Droz, 1968) and the pigment epithelium (Young and Bok, 1970), protein synthesis goes on continually in the nucleus, and in the cytoplasmic zone where ribosomes and RNA are concentrated.

Much of the protein formed in the cytoplasm is subsequently modified by the addition of carbohydrate, which serves a number of different functions. The oligosaccharide portion of opsin, for example, may act as a hydrophilic marker which keeps the protein oriented in the outer segment membrane (Heller and Lawrence, 1970). Carbohydrate-containing proteins (and lipids) of the cell membrane have their oligosaccharide components on the outside (Lehninger, 1968; Nicolson and Singer, 1974), where they may interact with extracellular ions, and serve as membrane recognition sites (e.g., for hormones, phagocytosis, or cell-to-cell adhesion).

The addition of carbohydrate to protein is controlled by many different enzymes, each representing a possible target for genetic lesion. There are two known mechanisms, both requiring as a first step enzymatic activation of monosaccharides by combination with a

nucleotide.   The first involves preassembly of part of the oligosaccharide chain on a lipid, dolichol phosphate, followed by
transfer to protein (Lennarz, 1975).   The other mechanism provides
for the addition of monosaccharides, one by one, in a definite
sequence, to form one or more simple or branched chains.   The
enzymes (glycosyl transferases) which transfer single sugars from
their nucleotide donors to protein acceptors are each specific for
the donor and acceptor molecules (O'Brien and Neufeld, 1972; Spiro,
1970; Roseman, 1970).   Glycoprotein glycosyl transferase enzymes
may occur in many locations within cells.

     In frog rods and cones, however, mannose glycoprotein trans-
ferases are confined to the myoid portion of the inner segment,
apparently in close association with the ribosomes (Young, 1974).
Much of the newly synthesized protein passes through the Golgi
complex after leaving the ribosomes (Young and Droz, 1968).   Experiments with labeled glucosamine suggest that the glycoprotein
transferase enzymes for this compound are located near the ribosomes and in the Golgi complex as well (Bok *et al.*, 1974; O'Brien
and Muellenberg, 1974).   In addition to its apparent content of
glycosyl transferases, the Golgi complex contains enzymes required
for the transfer of inorganic sulfate to many types of acceptor
molecules, including mucopolysaccharides (Young, 1973).   Rat visual
cells continually contribute to the renewal of the sulfated mucopolysaccharides in which their outer segments are embedded through
enzymatic pathways located in the inner segment of the cell (Ocumpaugh and Young, 1966; Hall *et al.*, 1965).   The pigment epithelium
may also contribute to the renewal of this material (Berman, 1964;
Young and Bok, 1976).

     The visual cells and pigment epithelium also renew their lip-
ids.   The frog pigment epithelial cells, for example, continually
replace a glycolipid in their oil droplets (Young and Bok, 1970).
Of particular importance are the phospholipids, which constitute a
major component of the membranes by which cells segregate the mul-
titude of metabolic activities required for their function and
survival.   The outer segments of the visual cells are a prime example of the critical importance of membranes in the economy of the
cell.

     Autoradiographic experiments in which glycerol, the structural
"backbone" of the phospholipid molecule, is supplied to frog visual
cells show that most of the glycerol is metabolized in the myoid
region of the inner segment (Bibb and Young, 1974b).   Choline and
inositol, two additional phospholipid constituents, are also primarily bound initially in the myoid region (Young and Basinger,
1975).   This is clearly the cell's major synthetic center for
renewal processes.

The complexity of lipid turnover is particularly evident when the renewal of fatty acids is analyzed. Radioactive palmitic acid is initially very heavily concentrated in the pigment epithelium (Bibb and Young, 1974a). Some of the fatty acid is used in the myoid region of the visual cells, probably in phospholipid synthesis, but a heavier incorporation is observed directly into the phospholipids of the rod and cone outer segment membranes. This indicates that not only are old phospholipid molecules continually replaced by new ones, but their fatty acid constituents are subsequently rapidly exchanged after the phospholipids are inserted in the membranes.

Another aspect of the visual cell renewal systems susceptible to genetic lesions are the carrier proteins which serve to solubilize, protect, and transport water-insoluble molecules through the aqueous media of the blood, tissue fluid and cells. Water-soluble plasma proteins play a major role in the transport of lipids. In the blood, vitamin A (retinol) is carried by a specific protein, retinol binding protein (RBP) which is synthesized in the liver (Muto et al., 1972; Kanai et al., 1968). Upon reaching the pigment epithelium, the retinol-RBP complex binds to a specific receptor on the cell membrane (Heller, 1975; Bok and Heller, 1976). Inside the cell, other specific proteins serve as carriers (Heller and Bok, 1976; Saari and Futterman, 1976; Wiggert et al., 1976). Phospholipids are moved around in cells by specific carrier proteins also (Wirtz, 1974).

Soon after synthesis, the proteins, glycoproteins and phospholipids produced in the myoid region of the visual cells begin to move to destinations in different parts of the cell, where they replace existing molecules of the same type. A considerable proportion of the protein, much of it now containing carbohydrate and possibly lipid, moves through the connecting cilium to reach the outer segment (Young, 1968). Here a striking difference between rod and cone renewal mechanisms is manifest. In rods, some of the protein spreads through the outer segment, but most of it becomes concentrated in new membranes which are continuously assembled at the base of the outer segment. No such localized accumulation is ever observed in cone outer segments. Instead, all of the renewal protein becomes scattered throughout the outer segment (Young, 1969a). The diffuse distribution of new protein molecules seems also to characterize the formation of cone outer segment membranes during cell differentiation (Ditto, 1975) and regeneration (unpublished work with C. E. Remé). Thus, both the biogenesis and renewal of rod and cone outer segment membranes proceed by somewhat different mechanisms.

Other rod-cone differences of a quantitative nature have been detected. Replacement of diffusely distributed protein (Bok and Young, 1972) and lipid (Bibb and Young, 1974a; Young and Basinger,

1975) occurs more rapidly in cone than in rod outer segments, but the replacement of mannose-containing protein is appreciably slower in cones (Young, 1974). In short, there is growing evidence of both qualitative and quantitative differences in rod and cone renewal mechanisms. These may prove to be involved in the differing responses of the two classes of visual cells in retinitis pigmentosa and allied degenerations.

In rods, repeated formation of new, disc-shaped membranes at the base of the outer segment displaces older membranes away from the base, towards the tip of the cell, where they are shed in little packets, surrounded by cell membrane (Young and Bok, 1969). The mechanism of shedding seems to involve the infolding of the outer membrane near the tip, dissecting from the end of the cell a few of the oldest membranes, and sealing off the tip of the cell in the process (Young, 1971b; Bok and Young, 1976). The pigment epithelium then phagocytizes the detached membranes and digests them intracellularly using its lysosomal enzymes. Any genetic defect affecting phagocytosis or intracellular digestion in the pigment epithelium would have very serious consequences for the rod visual cells.

EXAMPLES OF DISRUPTED RENEWAL SYSTEMS

An extreme example of an aberrant visual cell renewal system is evident in the RCS strain of rats. In these animals, the pigment epithelium fails completely to ingest the old rod outer segment membranes, which accumulate in a mass of debris at the tips of the rods (Herron *et al.*, 1969; Bok and Hall, 1971; LaVail and Mullen, 1976). Unlike the situation in RP and allied diseases, the rods do not reach full maturity in these rats before they begin to degenerate. However, the hereditary disease in RCS rats importantly demonstrates the principle that genetic disturbance of a renewal system can lead to visual cell death. In mammals, the entire outer segment of rods is replaced every one to two weeks (Young, 1967, 1971a). This is an indication that no such total failure of phagocytosis can occur in RP, where the onset of symptoms of degeneration does not occur until several years after birth.

It can be anticipated that a disturbance of fatty acid renewal mechanisms will seriously affect the visual cells. In rats, renewal of rod outer segments is modified when polyunsaturated fatty acids are withheld from the diet (Anderson *et al.*, 1974). One type of retinitis pigmentosa in man may also be due to a hereditary abnormality of fatty acid renewal. Refsum's syndrome is an autosomal recessive disease in which the defect is an absence or deficiency of the enzyme which oxidizes phytanic acid (a fatty acid quite similar to palmitic acid) leading to increased levels of phytanic acid in the blood (Baum *et al.*, 1965). The earliest symptom of the disease is night blindness, followed by the other symptoms of retinitis pigmentosa (Francois, 1975). Rods and cones degenerate, and the pigment epithelium, where present, is loaded with lipid deposits (Toussaint and Danis, 1971), apparently containing high levels of phytanic acid (Cumings, 1971).

The amino acid, taurine (which is not used for protein synthesis) is continually renewed in the visual cells of rats and frogs, apparently with the participation of the pigment epithelium (Young, 1969b). Cats fed a taurine-free casein diet develop plasma and retinal taurine deficiency with central retinal degeneration of the rods and cones (Hayes *et al.*, 1975; Schmidt *et al.*, 1975; Berson *et al.*, 1975). This appears to provide another example of disruption of a renewal system leading to visual cell death.

Vitamin A turnover serves as an additional case in point. This vitamin, a component of visual pigment, is continually renewed in visual cells (Bridges and Yoshikami, 1969; Hall and Bok, 1974). When it is withdrawn from the diet, the visual cells eventually degenerate (Dowling and Gibbons, 1961; Hayes, 1974), although storage of the vitamin in the pigment epithelium protects the viability of this renewal system until blood levels of the vitamin are exhausted (Dowling and Wald, 1958; Young and Bok, 1976).

Bassen-Kornzweig syndrome is a hereditary disease in which the primary defect seems to interfere with synthesis of the protein component of serum β-lipoproteins in the liver (Francois, 1975). The abnormality involves disturbances of lipid absorption and transport, including an inability to form chylomicrons. Because these serum lipoproteins normally transport lipids through the blood, plasma lipid fractions, including vitamin A, are markedly reduced in this disease (Gouras *et al.*, 1971). One of the abnormalities associated with the absence of the β-lipoproteins is degeneration of the visual cells, possibly due to a derangement in the renewal of lipids, including vitamin A (Gouras *et al.*, 1971; Harcourt, 1971). This is an example, then, of a genetic defect in a renewal system acting through an effect on carrier proteins.

SUMMARY AND CONCLUSION

The major theme developed in this manuscript is that retinitis pigmentosa and the progressive cone degenerations represent a family of diseases caused by different abnormal genes which provoke a similar effect in the retina--the degeneration of rods and cones. Because the defective genes do not prevent the differentiation of visual cells, but interfere with their long-term survival, it appears that they disrupt the normal operation of renewal systems. Furthermore, the differential effects on rods and cones in RP and related disease may well be due to intrinsic differences in renewal pathways in the two classes of visual cells.

The remarkable specialization of rods and cones, so successful from the standpoint of function, renders them particularly susceptible to damage from a wide variety of factors (Young, 1970). They are extremely sensitive, but very fragile. The continual operation of renewal systems, however, acts to heal injuries and prevent the accumulation of damage, so that normally the visual cells survive for a lifetime. Unfortunately, among all the cells in the visual system, they seem to be preferentially subject to genetically based failure of these renewal systems, so that in numerous genetic diseases and syndromes affecting vision, it is most often the rods and cones which degenerate.

Renewal processes depend upon a delicate balance between the production and degradation of molecules. In these hereditary retinal degenerations, the defective gene is almost certainly activated before birth, during cellular differentiation, but the visual cells do not die for several years or more. If the lesion disrupts renewal pathways, so that either synthesis or destruction is excessive or otherwise abnormal, why don't the cells degenerate immediately? It seems that the affected cells are able to adjust to the presence of the continued abnormal situation by attaining an altered steady-state, homeostatically maintained at an abnormal level. Cells may survive for extended periods while subjected to prolonged injuries by making adjustments of this sort (Trump and Arstila, 1971). However, if ultimately the continuing abnormality surpasses the capacities of alternative pathways to compensate, then the effects will finally be lethal, and the cell will degenerate.

It may sound axiomatic to suggest that retinitis pigmentosa and the allied cone degenerations could result from failure of rod and cone renewal mechanisms, because if the renewal process worked properly, the visual cells presumably would not degenerate. However, if we accept the usefulness of this general principle, at least as a working hypothesis, then it becomes clear that we should attempt to learn the details of these renewal processes so that ultimately we may understand how they can be disrupted. Then we will be in a position to discuss how such lesions might be treated.

ACKNOWLEDGEMENTS

Dr. Eliot Berson read an earlier draft of this manuscript, and offered several suggestions for its improvement. This assistance is gratefully acknowledged. The author's research is supported by United States Public Health Service Grants EY 00095 and EY 00444.

REFERENCES

Alström, C. H., Hallgren, B., Nilsson, L. B., and Asander, H. (1959) Retinal degeneration combined with obesity, diabetes mellitus and neurogenous deafness. *Acta Psychiat. Neurol. Scand.*, Suppl. 129, 34:1-35.

Anderson, R. E., Benolken, R. M., Dudley, P. A., Landis, D. J., and Wheeler, T. G. (1974) Polyunsaturated fatty acids of photoreceptor membranes. *Exp. Eye Res.* 18:205-213.

Archer, D. B., Krill, A. E., and Ernest, J. T. (1972) Choroidal vascular aspects of degenerations of the retinal pigment epithelium. *Trans. Ophthal. Soc. U. K.* 92:187-207.

Baum, J. L., Tannenbaum, M., and Kolodny, E. H. (1965) Refsum's syndrome with corneal involvement. *Amer. J. Ophthal.* 60:699-708.

Berman, E. R. (1964) The biosynthesis of mucopolysaccharides and glycoproteins in pigment epithelial cells of bovine retina. *Biochim. Biophys. Acta* 83:371-373.

Berson, E. L. (1973) Retinitis pigmentosa, the electroretinogram, and Mendel's laws. *Trans. Penn. Acad. Ophthal. Otolaryngol.*, 26:109-113.

Berson, E. L. (1975) Electrical phenomena in the retina, in "Adler's Physiology of the Eye" (R. A. Moses, ed.), pp. 453-499, C. V. Mosby Co., St. Louis.

Berson, E. L. (1976) Retinitis pigmentosa and allied retinal diseases: electrophysiological findings. *Trans. Amer. Acad. Ophthal. Otolaryngol.* (In press).

Berson, E. L., and Goldstein, E. B. (1970a) The early receptor potential in sex-linked retinitis pigmentosa. *Invest. Ophthal.* 9:58-63.

Berson, E. L., and Goldstein, E. B. (1970b) Early receptor potential in dominantly inherited retinitis pigmentosa. *Arch. Ophthal.* 83:412-420.

Berson, E. L., Gouras, P., and Gunkel, R. D. (1968a) Progressive cone-rod degeneration. *Arch. Ophthal.* 80:68-76.

Berson, E. L., Gouras, P., and Gunkel, R. D. (1968b) Progressive cone degeneration dominantly inherited. *Arch. Ophthal.* 80:77-83.

Berson, E. L., Gouras, P., Gunkel, R. D., and Myrianthopoulos, N. C. (1969a)   Rod and cone responses in sex-linked retinitis pigmentosa. *Arch. Ophthal.* 81:215-225.

Berson, E. L., Gouras, P., Gunkel, R. D., and Myrianthopoulos, N. C. (1969b) Dominant retinitis pigmentosa with reduced penetrance. *Arch. Ophthal.* 81:226-234.

Berson, E. L., Hayes, K. C., Rabin, A. R., Schmidt, S. Y., and Watson, G.   (1975)   Retinal degeneration in rats fed casein; II: Supplementation with methionine, cysteine, or taurine. *Invest. Ophthal.* 15:52-58.

Berson, E. L., and Howard, J. (1971) Temporal aspects of the electroretinogram in sector retinitis pigmentosa. *Arch. Ophthal.* 86:653-665.

Bibb, C., and Young, R. W. (1974a)   Renewal of fatty acids in the membranes of visual cell outer segments. *J. Cell Biol.* 61: 327-343.

Bibb, C., and Young, R. W.   (1974b) Renewal of glycerol in the visual cells and pigment epithelium of the frog retina. *J. Cell Biol.* 62:378-389.

Blodi, F. C. (1966)   The pathology of central tapeto-retinal dystrophy (hereditary macular degenerations).   *Trans. Amer. Acad. Ophthal. Otolaryngol.* 70:1047-1053.

Bok, D. (1966) RNA and DNA metabolism in rat photoreceptors. *Anat. Rec.* 154:320 (abstract).

Bok, D. (1970) The distribution and renewal of RNA in retinal rods. *Invest. Ophthal.* 9:516-523.

Bok, D., Basinger, S. F., and Hall, M. O. (1974) Autoradiographic and radiobiochemical studies on the incorporation of $(6-{}^3H)$ glucosamine into frog rhodopsin. *Exp. Eye Res.* 18:225-240.

Bok, D., and Hall, M. O. (1971) The role of the pigment epithelium in the etiology of inherited retinal dystrophy in the rat. *J. Cell Biol.* 49:664-682.

Bok, D., and Heller, J. (1976) Transport of retinol from the blood to the retina: An autoradiographic study of the pigment epithelial cell surface receptor for plasma retinol-binding protein. *Exp. Eye Res.* 22:395-402.

Bok, D., and Young, R. W. (1972) The renewal of diffusely distributed protein in the outer segments of rods and cones. *Vision Res.* 12:161-168.

Bok, D., and Young, R. W. (1976) Phagocytic properties of the retinal pigment epithelium in "The Retinal Pigment Epithelium" (K. M. Zinn and M. F. Marmor, eds.) Harvard University Press, Boston (In press).

Bridges, C. D. B., and Yoshikami, S. (1969) Uptake of tritiated retinaldehyde by the visual pigment of dark-adapted rats. *Nature* 221:275-276.

Carr, R. E. (1972) Symposium: Pigmentary retinopathy. Summing-up. *Trans. Ophthal. Soc. U. K.* 92:289-301.

Cherry, P. M. H. (1973) Usher's syndrome. *Ann. Ophthal.* 5:743-752.

Cockayne, E. A. (1936) Dwarfism with retinal atrophy and deafness. *Arch. Dis. Child.* 11:1-8.

Cogan, D. G. (1950) Pathology. *Trans. Amer. Acad. Ophthal. Otolaryngol.* 54:629-661.

Cumings, J. N. (1971) Inborn errors of metabolism in neurology (Wilson's disease, Refsum's disease and lipidoses). *Trans. Roy. Soc. Med.* 64:313-322.

Deutman, A. F. (1971) "The Hereditary Dystrophies of the Posterior Pole of the Eye" Charles C Thomas, Springfield.

Deutman, A. F. (1974) Macular dystrophies, in "Genetic and Metabolic Eye Disease" (M. F. Goldberg, ed.) pp. 367-429, Little Brown Co., Boston.

Ditto, M. (1975) A difference between developing rods and cones in the formation of outer segment membranes. *Vis. Res.* 15:535-536.

Dowling, J. E., and Gibbons, I. R. (1961) The effect of vitamin A deficiency on the fine structure of the retina, in "The Structure of the Eye" (G. Smelser, ed.) pp. 85-99, Academic Press, New York.

Dowling, J. E., and Wald, G. (1958) Vitamin A deficiency and night blindness. *Proc. Nat. Acad. Sci.* 44:648-661.

Droz, B. (1963) Dynamic condition of proteins in the visual cells of rats and mice as shown by radioautography with labeled amino acids. *Anat. Rec.* 145:157-168.

Francois, J. (1961) "Heredity in Ophthalmology" C. V. Mosby, St. Louis.

Francois, J. (1974a) L'hérédité des dégénérescences maculaires. *Ophthalmologica* 168:417-445.

Francois, J. (1974b) Ocular manifestations of the mucopolysaccharidoses. *Ophthalmologica* 169:345-361.

Francois, J., DeRouck, A., Verriest, G., DeLaey, J. J., and Cambie, E. (1974) Progressive generalized cone dysfunction. *Ophthalmologica* 169:255-284.

Gonin, J. (1903) Examen anatomique d'un oeil atteint de rétinite pigmentaire avec scotome zonulaire. *Anales d'Oculist.* 129:24-48.

Goodman, G., Ripps, H., and Siegel, I. M. (1963) Cone dysfunction syndromes. *Arch. Ophthal.* 70:214-231.

Gouras, P., Carr, R. E., and Gunkel, R. D. (1971) Retinitis pigmentosa in abetalipoproteinemia: effects of vitamin A. *Invest. Ophthal.* 10:784-793.

Hall, M.O., and Bok, D. (1974) Incorporation of (^{3}H) vitamin A into rhodopsin in light- and dark-adapted frogs. *Exp. Eye Res.* 18:105-117.

Hall, M. O., Ocumpaugh, D. E., and Young, R. W. (1965) The utilization of ^{35}S-sulfate in the synthesis of mucopolysaccharides by the retina. *Invest. Ophthal.* 4:322-329.

Harcourt, B. (1971) Inborn errors of metabolism. *Trans. Ophthal. Soc. U. K.* 90:117-126.

Hayes, K. C. (1974) Retinal degeneration in monkeys induced by deficiencies of vitamin E or A. *Invest. Ophthal.* 13:499-510.

Hayes, K. C., Carey, R. E., and Schmidt, S. Y. (1975) Retinal degeneration associated with taurine deficiency in the cat. *Science* 188:949-951.

Heller, J. (1975) Interactions of plasma retinol-binding protein with its receptor. Specific binding of bovine and human retinol binding protein to pigment epithelium cells from bovine eyes. *J. Biol. Chem.* 250:3613-3619.

Heller, J., and Bok, D. (1976) Transport of retinol from the blood to the retina: the involvement of high molecular weight lipoproteins as intracellular carriers. *Exp. Eye Res.* 22:403-410.

Heller, J., and Lawrence, M. A. (1970) Structure of the glycopeptide from bovine visual pigment 500. *Biochem.* 9:864-869.

Herron, W. L., Riegel, B. W., Myers, O. E., and Rubin, M. L. (1969) Retinal dystrophy in the rat--a pigment epithelial disease. *Invest. Ophthal.* 8:595-604.

Jay, B. (1972) Hereditary aspects of pigmentary retinopathy. *Trans. Ophthal. Soc. U. K.* 92:173-178.

Jay, B., and Bird, A. (1973) X-linked retinitis pigmentosa. *Trans. Amer. Acad. Ophthal. Otolaryngol.* 77:641-651.

Kanai, M., Raz, A., and Goodman, D. S. (1968) Retinol-binding protein: the transport protein for vitamin A in human plasma. *J. Clin. Invest.* 49:2025-2044.

Koenig, E. (1971) RNA synthesis in the rod cell of the rat. *Invest. Ophthal.* 10:794-799.

Kolb, H., and Gouras, P. (1974) Electron microscopic observations of human retinitis pigmentosa, dominantly inherited. *Invest. Ophthal.* 13:489-498.

Krill, A. E., Deutman, A. F., and Fishman, M. (1973) The cone degenerations. *Doc. Ophthal.* 35:1-80.

LaVail, M. M. (1973) Kinetics of rod outer segment renewal in the developing mouse retina. *J. Cell Biol.* 58:650-661.

LaVail, M. M., and Mullen, R. J. (1976) Role of the pigment epithelium in inherited retinal degeneration analyzed with chimeric mice and rats. *Exp. Eye Res.* 23:227-245.

Leber, T. (1915) Die Pigmentdegeneration der Netzhaut und die mit ihr verwandte Erkrankungen, in "Graefe-Saemisch Handbuch der gesamten Augenheilkunde (A. Wagenmann, ed.) Vol. 5, p. 1125, Wilhelm Engelmann, Leipzig.

Lehninger, A. L. (1968) The neuronal membrane. *Proc. Nat. Acad. Sci.* 60:1069-1080.

Lennarz, W. J. (1975) Lipid linked sugars in glycoprotein synthesis. *Science* 188:986-991.

Lucas, D. R. (1956) Retinitis pigmentosa. Pathological findings in two cases. *Brit. J. Ophthal.* 40:14-23.

Maraini, G., and Franguelli, R. (1962) Radioautographic investigations on nucleic acids and protein metabolism of the retina *in vitro. Ophthalmologica* 144:141-150.

Maraini, G., Franguelli, R., and Peralta, S. (1963) Studies on the metabolism of the retina and lateral geniculate nucleus. *Invest. Ophthal.* 2:567-570.

Mizuno, K, and Nishida, S. (1967) Electron microscopic studies of human retinitis pigmentosa. *Amer. J. Ophthal.* 63:791-803.

Muto, Y., Smith, J. E., Milch, P. O., and Goodman, D. S. (1972) Regulation of retinol-binding protein metabolism by vitamin A status in the rat. *J. Biol. Chem.* 247:2542-2550.

Nicolson, G. L., and Singer, S. J. (1974) The distribution and asymmetry of mammalian cell surface saccharides utilizing ferritin-conjugated plant agglutinins as specific saccharide stains. *J. Cell Biol.* 60:236-248.

Nover, A., and Schultz, B. (1960) Autoradiographische Untersuchung uber den Eiweissstoffwechsel in den Geweben und Zellen des Auges. *Graefe Arch. klin. exp. Ophthal.* 161:554-578.

O'Brien, P. J., and Muellenberg, C. G. (1974) The biosynthesis of rhodopsin *in vitro. Exp. Eye Res.* 18:241-252.

O'Brien, P. J., and Neufeld, E. F. (1972) Biosynthesis of glycoproteins. Glycosyltransferases, in "Glycoproteins" (A. Gottschalk, ed.) pp. 1170-1186, Elsevier, New York.

Ocumpaugh, D. E., and Young, R. W. (1966) Distribution and synthesis of sulfated mucopolysaccharides in the retina of the rat. *Invest. Ophthal.* 5:196-203.

Pearlman, J. T., Owen, W. G., and Brounley, D. W. (1974) Cone dystrophy with dominant inheritance. *Amer. J. Ophthal.* 77:293-303.

Roberts, J. A. F. (1970) "An Introduction to Medical Genetics," Butterworths, London.

Roseman, S. (1970) The synthesis of complex carbohydrates by multiglycosyltransferase systems and their potential function in intercellular adhesion. *Chem. Phys. Lipids* 5:270-297.

Saari, J. C., and Futterman, S. (1976) An intracellular retinol binding protein isolated from bovine retina: isolation and partial characterization. *Exp. Eye Res.* 22:425-433.

Schmidt, S. Y., Berson, E. L., and Hayes, K. D. (1975) Retinal degeneration in cats fed casein: I. Taurine deficiency. *Invest. Ophthal.* 15:47-52.

Schoenheimer, R. (1942) "The Dynamic State of Body Constituents," Harvard University Press, Boston.

Schultze, B., Apponi, G., and Nover, A. (1961) Autoradiographische Untersuchung mit H^3-Thymidin uber die Desoxyribonucleinsaure-Neubildung in den Geweben des Rattenauges. *Graefe Arch. Ophthal.* 163:130-138.

Sidman, R. L. (1961) Histogenesis of mouse retina studied with thymidine-H^3, in "The Structure of the Eye" (G. K. Smelser, ed.) pp. 487-506, Academic Press, New York.

Sloan, L. H., and Brown, D. (1962) Progressive retinal degeneration with selective involvement of the cone mechanism. *Amer. J. Ophthal.* 54:629-641.

Sorsby, A. (1972) Retina and choroid, in "Modern Ophthalmology" (A. Sorsby, ed.) Vol. 3, pp. 308-316, Butterworths, Washington.

Spiro, R. G. (1970) Glycoproteins. *Ann. Rev. Biochem.* 39:599-638.

Toussaint, D., and Danis, P. (1971) An ocular pathologic study of Refsum's syndrome. *Amer. J. Ophthal.* 72:342-347.

Trump, B. F., and Arstila, A. U. (1971) Cell injury and cell death, in "Principles of Pathobiology" (M. F. LaVia and R. B. Hill, eds.) pp. 9-95, Oxford University Press, New York.

Verhoeff, F. H. (1931) Microscopic observations in a case of retinitis pigmentosa. *Arch. Ophthal.* 5:392-407.

Wiggert, B. D., Bergsma, R., and Chader, G. J. (1976) Studies on the intracellular binding of retinol in the retina and pigment epithelium. *Exp. Eye Res.* 22:411-418.

Wirtz, K. W. A. (1974) Transfer of phospholipids between membranes. *Biochim. Biophys. Acta* 344:95-117.

Wolter, J. R. (1957) Retinitis pigmentosa. *Arch. Ophthal.* 57:539-553.

Young, R. W. (1965) Renewal of photoreceptor outer segments. *Anat. Rec.* 151:484 (abstract).

Young, R. W. (1966) Further studies on the renewal of photoreceptor outer segments. *Anat. Rec.* 154:446 (abstract).

Young, R. W. (1967) The renewal of photoreceptor cell outer segments. *J. Cell Biol.* 33:61-72.

Young, R. W. (1968) Passage of newly formed protein through the connecting cilium of retinal rods in the frog. *J. Ultrastruc. Res.* 23:462-473.

Young, R. W. (1969a) A difference between rods and cones in the renewal of outer segment protein. *Invest. Ophthal.* 8:222-231.

Young, R. W. (1969b) The organization of vertebrate photoreceptor cells, in "The Retina" (B. R. Straatsma, M. O. Hall, R. A. Allen, and F. Crescitelli, eds.) pp. 177-210, University of California Press, Los Angeles.

Young, R. W. (1970) Visual cells. *Sci. Amer.* 223:80-91.

Young, R. W. (1971a) The renewal of rod and cone outer segments in the rhesus monkey. *J. Cell Biol.* 49:303-318.

Young, R. W. (1971b) Shedding of discs from rod outer segments in the rhesus monkey. *J. Ultrastruc. Res.* 34:190-203.

Young, R. W. (1973) The role of the Golgi complex in sulfate metabolism. *J. Cell Biol.* 57:175-189.

Young, R. W. (1974) Metabolism of mannose by frog visual cells. Annual meeting of the Association for Research in Vision and Ophthalmology, Abstract #8, p. 34.

Young, R. W., and Basinger, S. (1975) Metabolism of choline and inositol by frog visual cells. Annual meeting of the Association for Research in Vision and Ophthalmology, Abstract #9, p. 59.

Young, R. W., and Bok, D. (1969) Participation of the retinal pigment epithelium in the rod outer segment renewal process. *J. Cell Biol.* 42:392-403.

Young, R. W., and Bok, D. (1970) Autoradiographic studies on the metabolism of the retinal pigment epithelium. *Invest. Ophthal.* 9:524-536.

Young, R. W., and Bok, D. (1976) Metabolism of the pigment epithelium, in "The Retinal Pigment Epithelium" (K. M. Zinn and
M. F. Marmor, eds.) Harvard University Press, Boston (In
press).

Young, R. W., and Droz, B. (1968) The renewal of protein in retinal rods and cones. *J. Cell Biol.* 39:169-184.

DISCUSSION OF THE PAPER

DR. SIEGEL: Do you think that the phagocytic processes are an active or a passive type?

DR. YOUNG: Studies on phagocytosis in other types of cells, such as neutrophils and histiocytes, indicate that energy is required for ingestion. Is that what you meant?

DR. SIEGEL: No. I meant, is the phagocytic process initiated by the tip of the rod pressing up against the pigment epithelium or does the pigment epithelium actively reach down and nibble off the rod?

DR. YOUNG: I think it is fair to say that there is still some doubt about this. If you consider the possibility first of all that the delicate cytoplasmic processes of the pigment epithelium are somehow capable of biting off a few discs, it is apparent that as they pulled them off, the end of the cell would be open, and the cytoplasm would leak out. However, the end of a rod always has an outer membrane covering it, and the shed discs are surrounded by an outer membrane. I think that the mechanism which I described and hoped to demonstrate through the pictures I showed is more likely. According to this alternative, the outer rod membrane folds in, dissects off the tip, and covers over the end of the cell at the same time. (We know that the outer membrane can fold in, because that is how the disc membranes are formed in the first place.) The pigment epithelium then recognizes that these shed discs should be scavenged.

DR. DOWLING: I would like to ask a question, Dick. It seems to me that if your idea that a defect in the renewal systems causes a disease like retinitis pigmentosa, it would seems to me that if you could stop the renewal process then one should observe quite rapidly the degeneration of visual cells. Now I know of the recent work from Baylor which shows that you can stop the renewal process in rods reasonably well by putting rats on an essentially fatty-acid free diet. Yet as I recall those results, the receptors don't tend to degenerate and you can record reasonably good potentials from those retinas. Would you care to comment on their studies?

DR. YOUNG: In the results that John is referring to, the animals were raised on lipid free diets--that is, a deficiency of essential fatty acids--but the cells managed to make their outer segment membranes; they insert other fatty acids in the place of the ones that are missing. In second and third generation animals raised on fat-free diets, the rods still make outer segments. So I don't think it is demonstrated that the renewal mechanisms are stopped. They are altered. They are influenced, but the cells make adjustments and manage to keep going.

DR. SREBRO: Have you looked for evidence of the renewal process like this anywhere else--in the brain--or is this completely unique to the retina?

DR. YOUNG: As far as I know, practically everything in the body is renewed, except the genetic material. In the brain, the phenomenon of axoplasmic flow, which is a renewal process, has been well known since the 1940's. I have mainly been concerned with renewal systems in rods and cones. The fact that most of the constituents of our bodies are continually replaced is something to think about. We are sitting here today with different bodies than we had a couple of years ago.

DR. DOWLING: Fortunately!

RAT MODEL FOR HEREDITARY RETINAL DEGENERATION

Yin-Lok Lai and Albert M. Jonas

Section of Comparative Medicine
Yale University School of Medicine
New Haven, Connecticut 06510

INTRODUCTION

Inherited retinal degeneration affects man (Verhoeff, 1931; Cogan, 1950), dogs (Parry, 1953; Lucas, 1954; Barnett, 1962), mice (Keeler, 1924; Hopkins, 1927; Cohrs, 1933; Bruckner, 1951; Transley, 1951; Sorsby et al., 1954; LaVail and Sidman, 1974), and rats (Bourne et al., 1938; Lucas et al., 1955; Dowling and Sidman, 1962). Due to the complexity of the disease and the difficulties of obtaining human retinal tissue for studies, human hereditary retinal disorders have been very inadequately described, and much of the information concerning the subject is derived from investigations of animal models.

Two rodent models have been widely used for the studies of hereditary retinal degeneration: the RCS rat and the rd mouse. Hereditary retinal degeneration was first described by Bourne et al. (1938) and was due to an autosomal recessive gene (Bourne and Gruneberg, 1939; Lucas et al., 1955). It was first detected in 12 day old newborn rat retinas as the appearance of extracellular lamellae between developing rods and pigment epithelium. This was followed by further disorganization of photoreceptor outer segments by 18 days of age, degeneration of photoreceptor nuclei by day 22, and changes in the pigment epithelium by day 40. Inner segments, nuclei and synaptic processes of photoreceptor cells disappeared entirely by 60 days (Dowling and Sidman, 1962). Pigment epithelium of the RCS rat fails to ingest the outer segments of the photoreceptors, and cause accumulation of outer segment material with resulting degeneration of the photoreceptor cells (Herron et al., 1969; Bok and Hall, 1971; LaVail et al., 1972). The primary lesion in the retinal dystrophy of the RCS rat is thus at the level of pigment epithelium. Retinal dystrophy in mice has also been extensively investigated (Keeler, 1924; Hopkins, 1927;

Cohrs, 1933; Bruckner, 1951; Tansley, 1951; Karli, 1952; Sorsby *et al.*, 1954; LaVail and Sidman, 1974). Degeneration begins ten days after birth and by 21 days most of the rod layer has vanished. Retinal degeneration in mice begins before differentiation of the retina is completed and is thus an arrest of normal retinal development.

Retinitis pigmentosa in man differs from the RCS rat model in that degeneration in RCS rats is due to a failure of phagocytosis by pigment epithelium, whereas phagocytosis in affected human retinal pigment epithelium seems normal (Kolb and Gouras, 1974). Furthermore, unlike the retinal disorder in rd mice, retinitis pigmentosa is rarely manifested at birth, but rather becomes apparent in childhood. Most patients have years of normal retinal function before the appearance of degeneration of photoreceptors and evidence of retinal aplasia has not been documented in retinitis pigmentosa.

Apparent differences between existing animal models and retinitis pigmentosa and the difficulties of obtaining human retinal tissue for research have stimulated exploration for new animal models which would increase understanding, treatment, and prevention of retinitis pigmentosa. We have discovered a new form of spontaneous bilateral retinal degeneration in Wag/Rij rats. It is characterized by early onset, and a slowly progressive course. Degeneration appears to begin in the photoreceptor cell body and only secondarily affects its outer segment. Furthermore, the phagocytic activity of the pigment epithelium remains intact. Endstage lesions include disappearance of photoreceptor cells, migration of the pigment epithelium and disorganization of the affected retina. These lesions closely resemble those of retinitis pigmentosa (Lai *et al.*, 1975).

This chapter reviews briefly our work on the characterization of the retinal degeneration in Wag/Rij rats and gives speculations for future research.

MATERIALS AND METHODS

Breeding pairs of inbred Wag/Rij rats were initially obtained from the Radiobiological Institute T.N.O. (H.S.R.) Rijswijk, Netherlands, and a small colony was established at Yale by brother x sister matings. They were housed in a controlled environment room within a barrier facility and fed rat chow and hyperchlorinated water (9 p.p.m.) ad libitum. Once a breeder pair was established, their location remained constant, and they were exposed to the same light intensity throughout life. Weanling rats were handled in an identical manner. Ambient lighting was provided by ceiling-mounted 40 watt fluorescent lamps regulated on a 12 hours on, 12 hours off cycle. Approximate reflected light intensities were measured as 32 footcandles at cages positioned on the top of each rack, 5 footcandles at the middle shelf, and 1 footcandle at cages located on the bottom shelf.

More than 100 Wag/Rij rats of both sexes from 2 weeks to 32 months of age were used to study the development of the retinal degeneration. Twenty-eight male Fischer rats from 1 to 10 months of age and six male DA rats from 3 to 8 months of age were used in this study as controls.

Animals were anesthetized and euthanatized by intraperitoneal injection of sodium pentobarbital. Rats were perfused through the left ventricle and aorta with 2-4% glutaraldehyde in 0.1 M phosphate buffer, pH 7.4, under continuous pressure of lower than 80 mm Hg for about 20 minutes. Eyes were dissected and immersed in fixative for two hours at room temperature and washed briefly in 0.134 M phosphate buffer. Eye cups were postfixed for two to three hours in 1% osmium tetroxide buffered with 0.1 M phosphate. Fixed eye cups were then dehydrated in graded ethanols, cleared in propylene oxide, and embedded in Spurr's medium (Spurr, 1969).

The embedded eye cups were halved through the optic head posterio-anteriorly, and 1 μ sections of the hemispheres of the eye cup, including a full length of the retina between two sides of ora serrata and the optic disc, were prepared with glass knives and stained with Azur 11-methylene blue (Richardson *et al.*, 1960) for light microscopy. Selected areas were prepared for electron microscopy and placed on bare copper grids. Ultra-thin sections were double stained with uranyl acetate (Gibbons and Grimstone, 1960) and lead citrate (Reynolds, 1963).

RESULTS

Progression of the Disease

The retinas of 1 month old Wag/Rij rats were well developed, and matched those in control normal rats except for a few scattered degenerated photoreceptors. By 3 months of age, increased numbers of degenerating cells were found in outer and inner nuclear layers (Fig. 1). Changes became more widespread by 6 months of age and the thickness of the outer nuclear (photoreceptor) layer was reduced from about 12 cells to about eight cells per column. Photoreceptor degeneration progressed during the next several months and advanced degeneration was seen in most rats by 12 months (Fig. 1 insert).

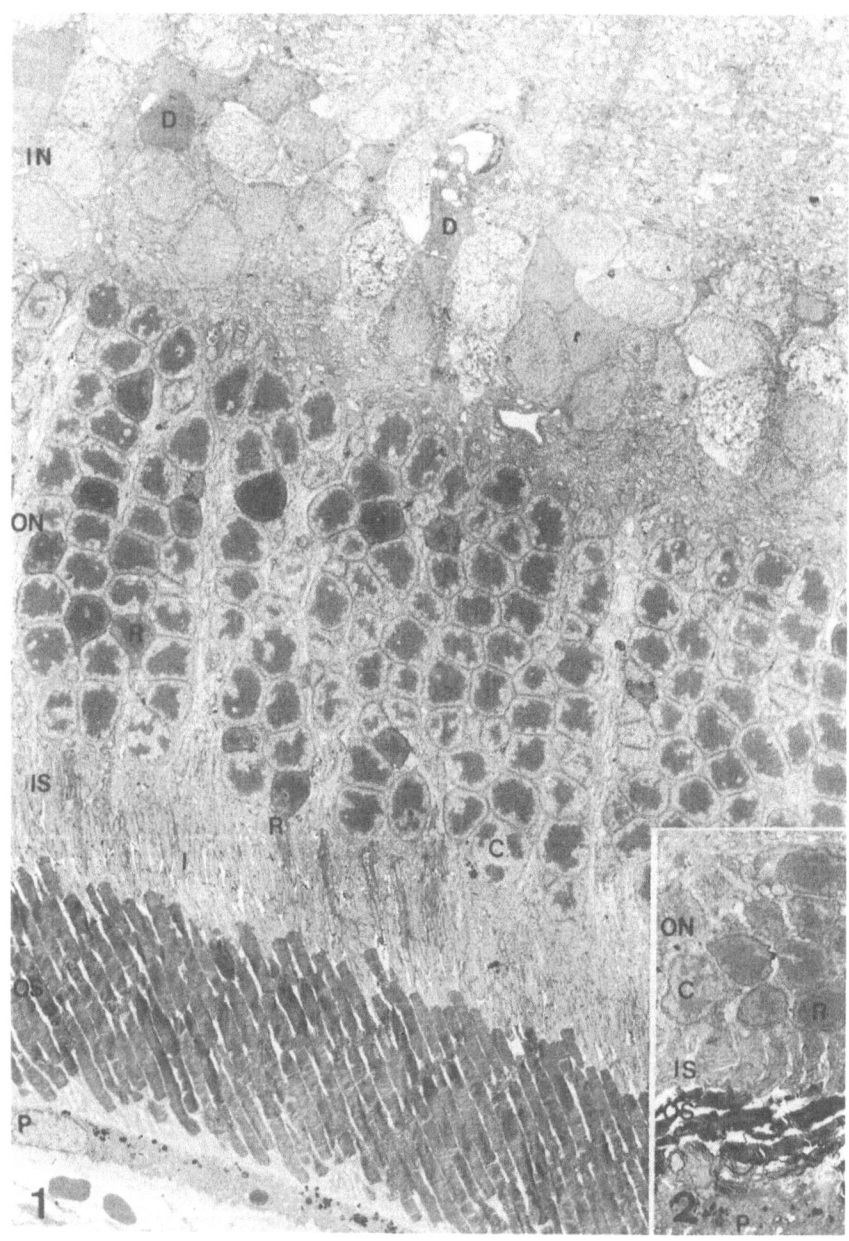

Figures 1 and 2

The absolute number of degenerated photoreceptor cells, and the ratio of degenerated photoreceptor cells to the structurally normal photoreceptor cells in an affected retina was not always related to the severity of loss of photoreceptors in the outer nuclear layer. Early in the disease, a small number of degenerated photoreceptor cells were found among structurally normal photoreceptor cells (Fig. 1). The length of photoreceptor inner and outer segments was progressively reduced, which matched the severity of loss of photoreceptor cells in the outer nuclear layer. By the age of 12 months the thickness of the outer nuclear (photoreceptor) layer was reduced to about four or five cells per column. Most photoreceptor cells in the affected retina became more and diffusely chromatophilic, and their inner and outer segments were considerably shorter and irregularly oriented. It looked, therefore, as if most of the photoreceptor cells at this stage of the disease were probably undergoing degeneration (Fig. 2).

Cytopathology of the Disease

The characteristics and progression of degeneration are similar in all cells regardless of time of onset. We have recognized

---

FIGURE 1. Three-month-old Wag/Rij rat. Numerous scattered degenerated rod cells (R) with increased electron density and shrinkage of cell body are present primarily in the left hand side of the micrograph. The variation in electron density suggests stage of degeneration. A cone cell (C) contains several electron dense juxtanuclear cytoplasmic inclusions in the lower right hand side of the micrograph. The outer nuclear layer (ON) has thinned to about 8 to 10 cells per column. Two degenerated cells (D) are present in the inner nuclear layer (IN). X 1800

FIGURE 2. Twelve-month-old Wag/Rij rat. This lesion has lost most of its photoreceptors. The outer nuclear layer (ON) has thinned to about 3 or 4 cells per column. Photoreceptor inner segments (IS) and outer segments (OS) are shorter and disorganized. Surviving rod cells have higher electron density and probably are undergoing degeneration. A small pile of disintegrated outer segment is shown in the lower left hand side of the micrograph. X 1800

[A complete explanation of all figure abbreviations is given at the end of the text.]

two forms of degeneration in photoreceptor cells in Wag/Rij rat
retinas: the degeneration with shrinkage of the cell body and
degeneration with swelling of the cell body. Alterations are also
observed in the synaptic terminal and inner segment of the affected
photoreceptor cell and they precede changes in the outer segment.

Rod Cells. Degeneration with shrinkage of the cell body was
observed exclusively in the rod cells (Fig. 1). At early stages,
the affected rod cell had a normal structure, but a somewhat
increased intensity of staining. This is correlated ultrastruc-
turally with an increased electron density in the cytoplasmic and
nuclear matrix. The electron density of the chromatin mass in the
affected nucleus is, however, not increased initially. In the
inner segment, the Golgi apparatus was slightly dilated and the
mitochondria are smaller. Besides the occasional appearance of
intramitochondrial granules, the volume of mitochondria in affected rod spherules is smaller than normal. When the intensity of
staining further increases, the structure of the affected rod cell
becomes less distinguishable and more homogeneous. The increase
of intensity of staining is followed by cellular shrinkage, which
is sometimes accompanied with appearance of narrow clear space
around the degenerated rod cell. In advanced stages degenerated
rod cells become angular and they disintegrate into fragments.

Cone Cells. There was previously controversy as to whether
or not cone cells are present in rat retinas. Their presence,
however, is well documented.

Menner (1928) and Walls (1936) described cone nuclei as large
and ovoid with numerous small masses of chromatin, and their cells
were typical cones, except for the absence of a differentiated
ellipoid. Later, Sidman (1958) also confirmed that cone cells in
the rat retina were similar to those of other mammals, both in
appearance and in histochemical staining properties. The ultrastructure of synaptic triads in the rat retina was recently found
to be identical with cone pedicles in other mammal retinas (Ladman,
1958; Dubin, 1970; Sosula and Glow, 1970; Leure-Dupree, 1974).
Electronmicroscopy has also observed some photoreceptor inner and
outer segments in the rat retina which have characteristics of
cones (Dowling, 1967). Besides this morphological evidence, it
had been observed electrophysiologically that a second type of
receptor contributed to the electroretinogram (ERG) of the light
adapted rat retina. It differed from a rod in absolute threshold,
spectral sensitivity, and speed of response (Green, 1971).

In Wag/Rij rats, degeneration with swelling of the cell body
was observed exclusively in the cone cells (Figs. 3, 4, 5). There
was a conspicuous presence of some chromatophilic particles in the
cytoplasm of the cone cells. These particles were irregular in
outline and had a highly heterogeneous interior consisting of

extremely electron dense, membranous components of varying sizes and shapes. They were usually limited by a single membrane. These particles were mostly distributed in the juxtanuclear cytoplasm of the affected cone cells. The staining intensity of the affected cone cells decreased progressively and cytoplasmic and nuclear volumes were increased progressively. The swollen cytoplasm became homogeneous and lost its normal reticulated appearance. In the later stages of degeneration, the nuclear chromatin appeared to be dissolved and the nucleus of the affected cone cell gradually faded. Similar changes were found in the synaptic pedicle of the affected cone cell (Fig. 6).

The extent of cone cell degeneration varied from animal to animal, and was not always related to the extent of degeneration in rod cells.

Retinal Pigment Epithelium. The morphology of the retinal pigment epithelium in Wag/Rij rats is identical with that described by Dowling and Gibbons (1962) in other strains of rats. Fragments of phagocytized photoreceptor outer segments are demonstrable in Wag/Rij rat retinas (Lai *et al.*, 1975).

Some ultrastructural alterations have been observed in the retinal pigment epithelium of Wag/Rij rats during the course of degeneration. Numerous phagosomes, lysosomes, lipofuscin granules and residual bodies accumulated in the cytoplasm of the retinal pigment epithelium. The absolute number and the relative ratio of each category of these particles vary widely. The retinal pigment epithelium of the young Wag/Rij rats predominantly contains lysosomes (Fig. 7). More lipofuscin granules are found in the pigment epithelium of the older animals with widespread or severe retinal degeneration (Figs. 8 ,9). The pigment epithelium in the advanced degenerated retinas which lost most or all photoreceptor cells contains predominantly residual bodies (Fig. 10). The mitochondria in the affected retinal pigment epithelium are also progressively smaller and show higher electron density. The endoplasmic reticulum, especially the rough-surfaced endoplasmic reticulum, the free ribosomes as well as the electron density of the cytoplasmic matrix, are gradually increased (Figs. 7, 8, 9). There are also ultrastructural alterations in the basal surface of the affected pigment epithelium, which include a considerable increase of the depth of basal infoldings, and the filling of basal infoldings by electron dense granular and/or fibrillar substance resembling basement membrane material. A large number of disintegrated photoreceptor outer segments were present between the distal ends of the photoreceptor outer segments and the apical surface of the pigment epithelium of the advanced degenerated Wag/Rij retinas over 12 months of age (Fig. 11). Despite the presence of large numbers of disintegrated photoreceptor outer segments in the place, there is

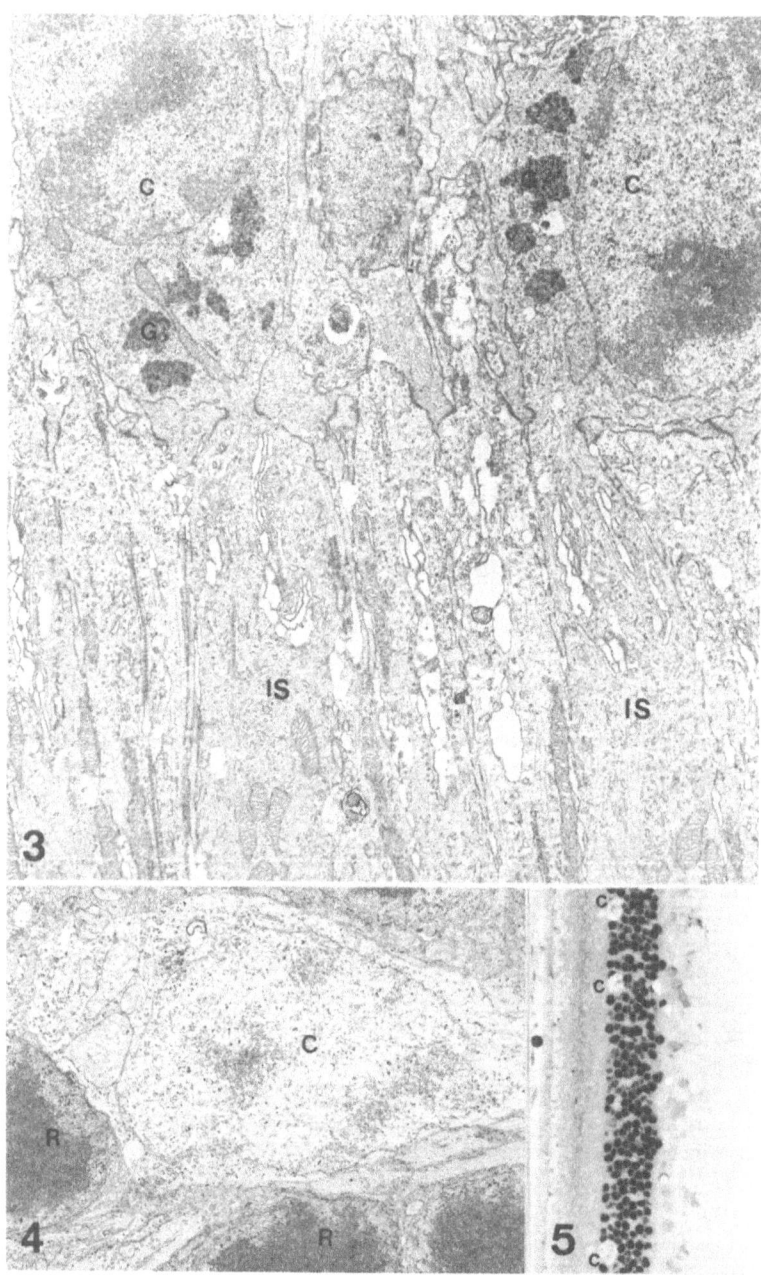

Figures 3, 4, and 5

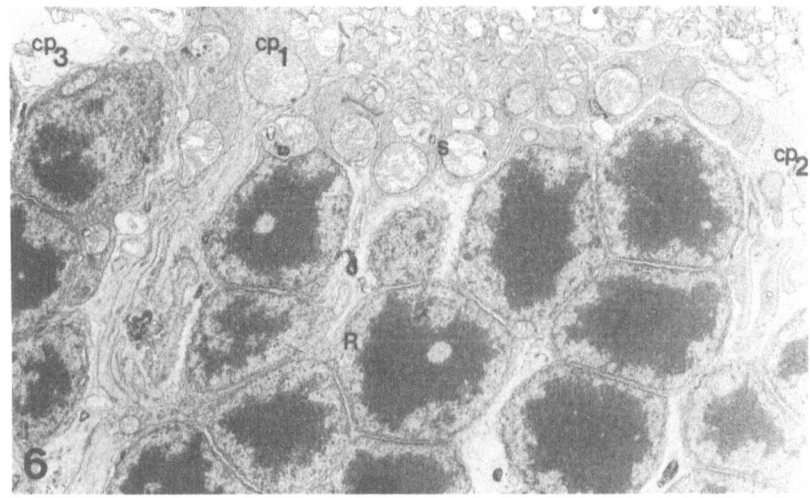

FIGURE 6. Three cone pedicles (cp) are shown in this micrograph.
The cp 1 is structurally normal; the cp 2 has lower electron
density than normal; the cp 3 is degenerated. X 5400

FIGURE 3. Two degenerating cone cells (C) are shown in this micrograph. Electron dense, juxtanuclear located, cytoplasmic
inclusions are present in these two cone cells. X 5400

FIGURE 4. A degenerated cone cell is shown in this micrograph.
This cone cell has very low electron density. Nuclear chromatin appears to be dissolved. X 5400

FIGURE 5. Three swollen cone cells (C) are shown in this micrograph. These cone cells stain palely. Their swollen inner
segments and synaptic pedicle are also distinguishable in
this micrograph. X 150

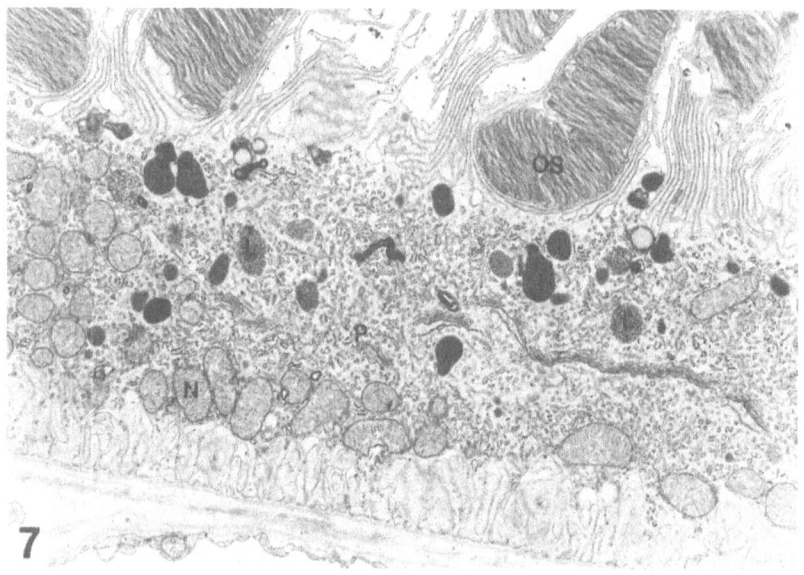

FIGURE 7. A pigment epithelial cell from a 6 month old Wag/Rij
rat retina. The cytoplasmic inclusions in this cell are predominantly lysosomes (L). X 9200

FIGURE 8. A pigment epithelial cell from a 14 month old Wag/Rij
rat. It contains a large number of cytoplasmic particles
which are irregular in outline and have a highly heterogeneous
interior consisting of dense bodies of varying sizes. These
particles are probably lipofuscin granules (Lf). X 9200

FIGURE 9. A pigment epithelial cell from a 14 month old Wag/Rij
rat. This contains fewer lipofuscin granules (Lf). An increase
in depth of basal infoldings (E 1) is shown in the lower left
hand side. The basal infoldings in the lower right hand side
are normal. X 9200

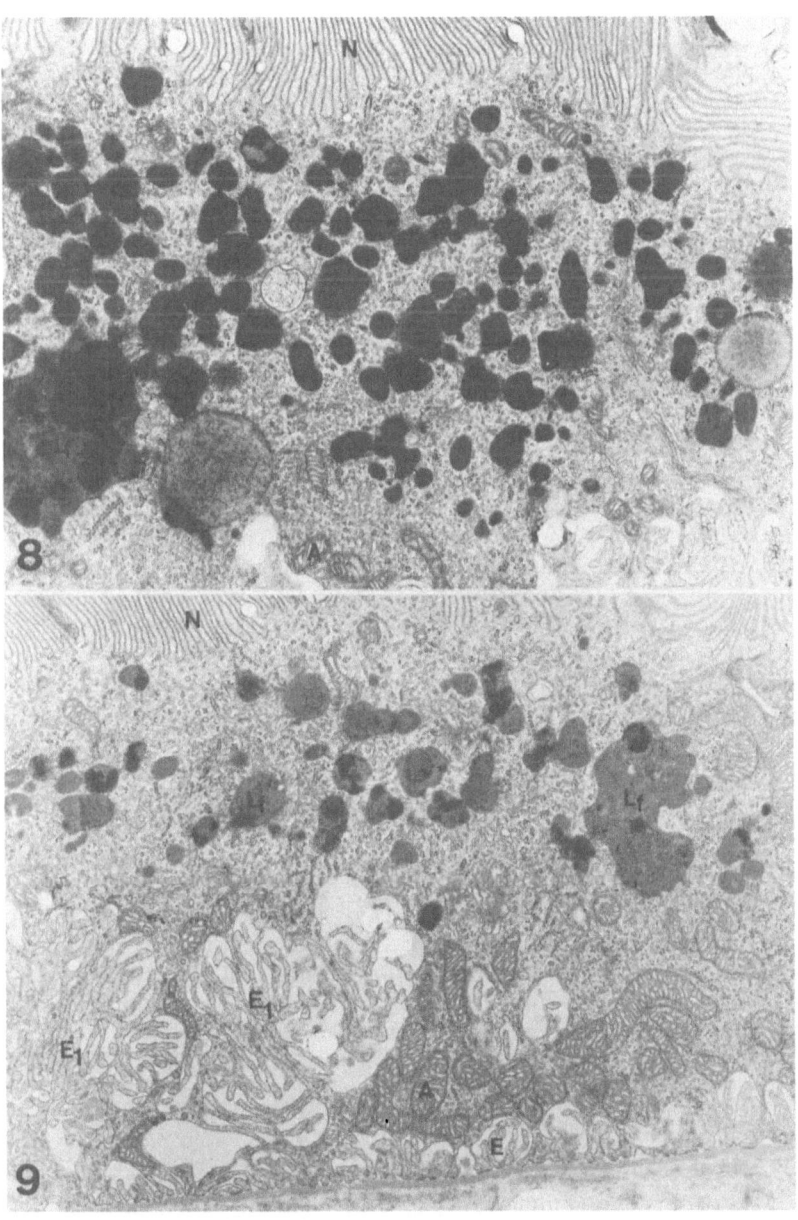

Figures 8 and 9

no evidence suggesting an increase in number of either lysosomes
or phagocytized lamellar material in that pigment epithelium.

In the endstage retina two distinctive types of cells are
found in the affected pigment epithelium (Fig. 10). The first type
closely resembles the normal pigment epithelium, but is somewhat
larger. The second type is a smaller, star-shaped chromatophilic
cell which contains little or no electron dense cytoplasmic particles. Instead of normally apical microvilli and basal infoldings,
the second type cell projects dendrites to all directions. At the
end of each dendrite a few microvilli branch to make contact with
neighboring cells.

The Effect of Ambient Light on the Development
of Retinal Lesions

Wag/Rij rats were housed in a controlled environment under a
light intensity of 5 footcandles, which should not cause retinal
damage. Five animals were euthanatized at 3 months of age for
pathological evaluation. Extensive degeneration was observed in
the outer nuclear (photoreceptor) layer and the inner layer (Fig.
12), which is identical with those observed in other Wag/Rij rats.
Dim light conditions lowered the speed of retinal degeneration
significantly, but failed to prevent the development of the
disease.

FIGURE 10. Two types of cells are observed in this pigment epithelium. The cell in the upper left hand side closely resembles
the normal pigment epithelium and contains predominantly
small, very electron dense, residual bodies (arrows). Two
smaller, stellate-shaped cells which contain no electron dense
cytoplasmic particles are in the lower right hand side of this
micrograph.

FIGURE 11. Fourteen-month-old Wag/Rij rat. A large number of disintegrated outer segments (Od) are on the apical surface of
the pigment epithelium. The pigment epithelium contains normal numbers of lysosomes (L). X 250

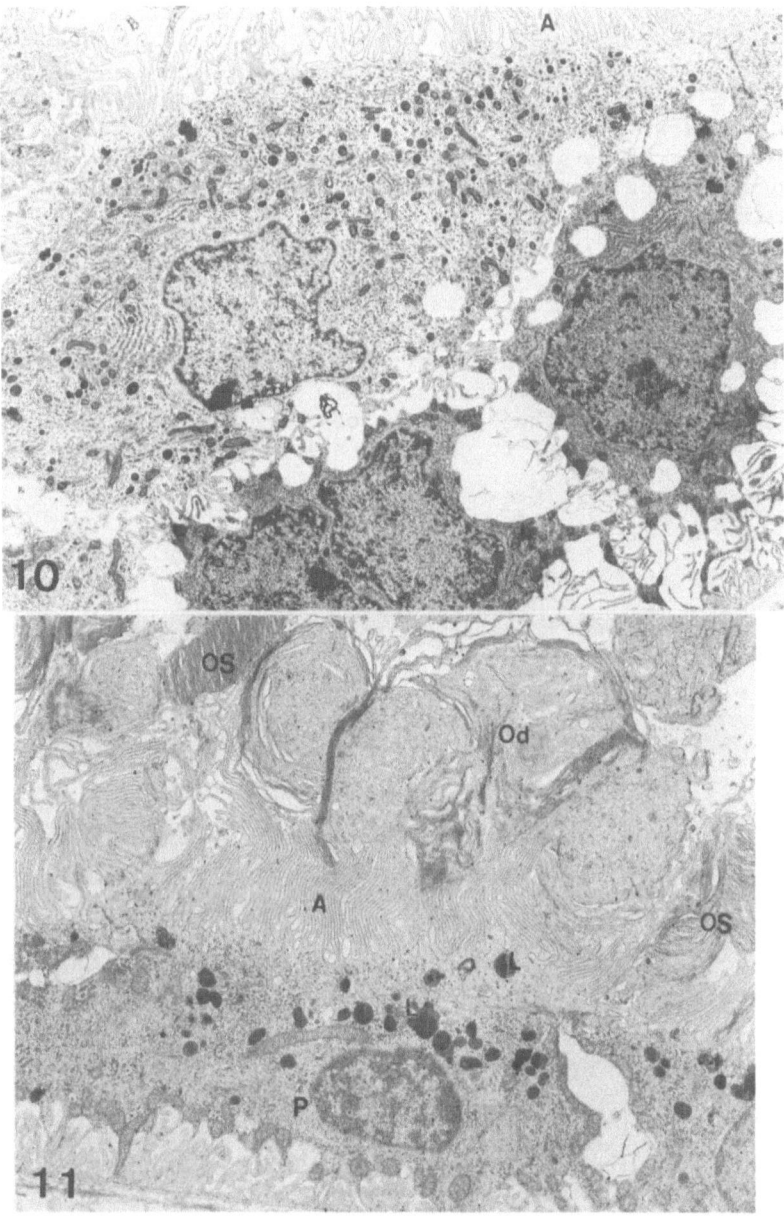

Figures 10 and 11

Inheritability of the Retinal Degeneration

F1 hybrids from albino Wag/Rij and nonalbino DA parents were studied. Eighteen F1 hybrids were euthanatized at 9 months of age for pathological evaluation. This experiment revealed that the thickness of the retina and the number of photoreceptor cells in the hybrids were substantially reduced due to identical cytopathological changes (Fig. 13).

DISCUSSION

Retinal degeneration in Wag/Rij rats is very characteristic in a comparative pathological sense. It is expressed in three principle features: the presence of a considerable number of degenerated photoreceptor cells, followed by a marked loss of

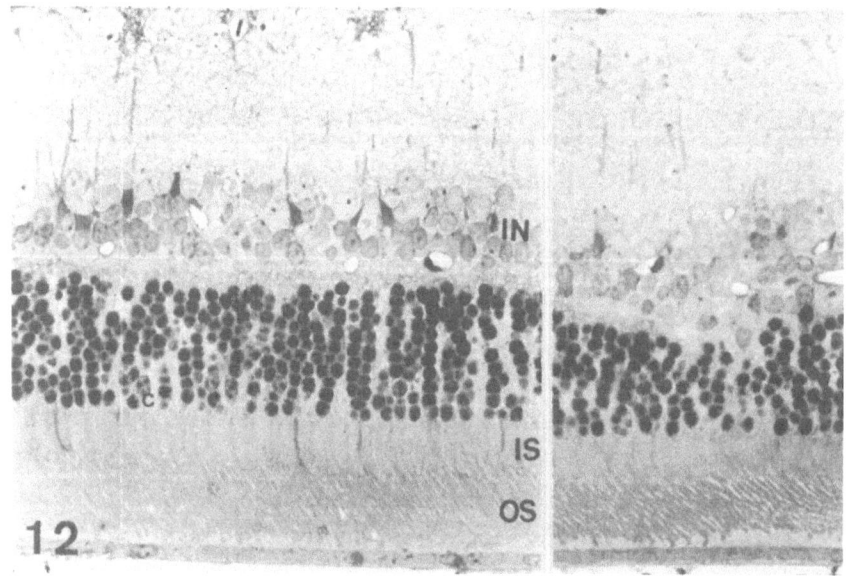

FIGURE 12. Three-month-old Wag/Rij rats raised under a light intensity of 5 footcandles. The outer nuclear layer of this retina is slightly thinner than normal and has about 8 to 10 cells per column. A large number of chromatophilic degenerated cells are present in inner and outer nuclear layers of this retina. A focal lesion is shown in the right hand side of the picture. X 250

photoreceptor cells in the affected retinas; the effect of the disease on cells in the inner nuclear layer; and the progression of retinal degeneration accompanied by marked changes in pigment epithelium. The possibility of environmental influence on the development of the retinal degeneration is very remote, since other strains of rats raised in identical animal care units and provided with the same sources of food, water, and illumination, did not develop retinal degeneration.

The damaging effect of the visible light on the retina has been well documented. The pathological mechanism of light damaged retina has been related to the nature of light sources, and duration of light exposure. High intensity incandescent light can cause rapid pyknosis of the visual cells and severe damage to the pigment epithelium (Noell *et al.*, 1966; Kuwabara and Gorn, 1968). High intensity fluorescent light can cause degeneration of the outer segments of the receptor cells first, then the synaptic terminals of the receptors, and finally involve the receptor cell bodies (Kuwabara and Gorn, 1968). Continuous low levels of illumination can cause a selective destruction of photoreceptor cells (O'Steen, 1970; O'Steen and Anderson, 1971, 1972). In this study, Wag/Rij rats were never exposed to light intensities over 35 footcandles or to continuous room illumination over 12 hours at a time.

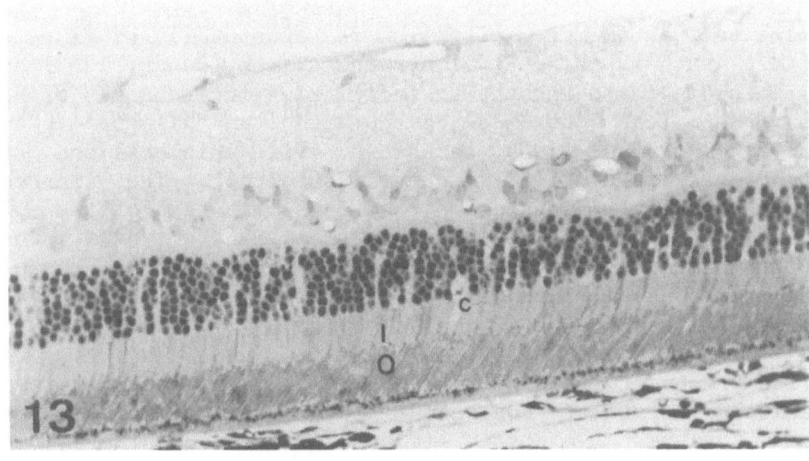

FIGURE 13. Nine-month-old Wag/Rij X DA F1 hybrid. This retina is heavily pigmented and is thinner than normal. Large numbers of degenerated photoreceptor cells are present in this retina. A degenerated cone cell with swelling of the cell body is shown in the center of the picture. X 150

The histopathology of the retinal degeneration in Wag/Rij rats also differs from those retinal lesions caused by light damage, since it is far more extensive and involves neurons in the inner retinal layers. Experimental Wag/Rij rats raised under very low light intensity (5 footcandles on the floor of the cages) developed identical retinal lesions at 3 months of age. All of these findings support our assumption that the retinal degeneration in Wag/Rij rats is a spontaneous disease and is not caused by the damaging effect of visible light.

The precise inheritance of the retinal disease in Wag/Rij rats has not been established; however, initial matings of Wag/Rij rats (albino) to pigmented DA rats showed extensive retinal degeneration among pigmented F1 hybrids which was identical to those of the Wag/Rij rats. This initial finding suggests that the gene for the retinal degeneration is separate from the gene for pigmentation and that degeneration is inherited as an autosomal dominant trait.

The progressive changes in the ultrastructure of the pigment epithelium during the course of retinal degeneration is striking. The changes in mitochondria, endoplasmic reticulum, and ribosomes demonstrate a profound alteration in metabolic activities of the pigment epithelium during the course of the disease. It is very possible that certain metabolic and/or functional alterations might occur before the morphological changes become detectable. If this is the case then the pigment epithelium might play a role in the retinal degeneration in Wag/Rij rats.

The retinal pigment epithelium is structurally similar to the choroid plexus in the central nervous system (Cohen, 1963) and the basal infoldings are thought to facilitate interchanges of metabolites between the choroidal circulation and pigment epithelium (Bernstein and Pease, 1959; Bernstein, 1961; Wislocki and Ladman, 1955; Yamada et al., 1958; Cohen, 1960, 1961). The increase in depth of basal infoldings suggests a metabolic need of the pigment epithelium to increase the interchanges of metabolites. This would be coincidental to changes in cellular organelles in the pigment epithelium. The filling of basal infoldings in man is thought to be an age related change (Hogan et al., 1971).

The presence of disintegrated photoreceptor outer segments at the apical surface of the retinal pigment epithelium is a very unusual feature. Two possibilities have been considered relating to this phenomenon: (1) an increase of the amount of outer segment material available for removal due to either an increase of biosynthesis of photoreceptor outer segments or widespread degeneration of photoreceptors which is beyond the phagocytic capacity of the pigment epithelium; or (2) the efficiency of phagocytosis in the pigment epithelium is reduced for unknown reasons. We have no information at hand to prove the possibility of an increase of biosynthesis of outer segments in Wag/Rij rats. Kuwabara and Gorn (1968) demonstrated an increase of lysosome and phagosome populations in the light damaged retina following widespread destruction of the photoreceptor and accumulation of an extraordinary amount of photoreceptor outer segment for removal. Their experiment demonstrated that the pigment epithelium is able to phagocytize an increased amount of photoreceptor outer segments if the pigment epithelium is not damaged. However, there is no evidence suggesting an increase in number of phagosomes in the affected pigment epithelium of Wag/Rij rats. It is assumed that either the reduced efficiency of phagocytosis in the pigment epithelium or the change in the outer segment membranes which caused them not to be ingested in the normal way might be responsible for the changes.

The demonstration of ultrastructural alteration in the pigment epithelium of Wag/Rij rats during the course of retinal degeneration implicates the possibility of interactions between the pigment epithelium and the photoreceptor cells.

Retinal degeneration in Wag/Rij rats also affects the cells of the inner nuclear layer, particularly the Muller's cells. The Muller's cells have been demonstrated to contain oxidative enzymes (Kuwabara and Cogan, 1960). These cells are the site of biosynthesis and storage of glycogen (Kuwabara and Cogan, 1961), and are thought to funnel nutritional material to the retinal neurons (Sjostrand, 1960; Cogan, 1962). The pathogenesis of the disease in Wag/Rij rats might be more complicated than just an interaction between the pigment epithelium and the photoreceptor. It is probable that the Muller's cells also play a role in the pathogenesis of the disease.

Characterization of the retinal lesions should be the single most important and essential work which would contribute to the understanding of the disease. Therefore, more extensive quantitative and sequential studies should be carried out to refine the present knowledge of the disease and to explore possible clues of interactions among retinal elements, i.e., the rod-cone interaction, photoreceptor-Muller cell interaction, and photoreceptor-pigment epithelium interaction.

CONCLUSIONS

The disorder in Wag/Rij rats is a spontaneous, bilateral retinal degeneration. It is characterized by an early onset, slowly progressive degeneration of the photoreceptor cells leading to destruction of the retina. Degeneration affects both rod cells and cone cells, and to a lesser degree the cells in the inner nuclear layer. The remarkable alterations in the retinal pigment epithelium during the course of the disease suggest a profound change in metabolism and function of the pigment epithelium and implicate a possibility of interaction between the pigment epithelium and the photoreceptors. Since degenerated cells have also been observed in the inner nuclear layers, there is a possibility that Muller's cells are involved in the retinal degeneration. Controlled experiments have demonstrated that the disease is not induced by light damaging effects of the retina, and initial breeding experiments suggest that the disease is inheritable, probably as an autosomal dominant trait.

The retinal degeneration in Wag/Rij rats is a new, unique system and it is a potentially very useful animal model of retinitis pigmentosa.

ACKNOWLEDGEMENTS

This investigation was supported by Public Health Service grants USPHS RR 00393-09, USPHS RR 05358-14, USPHS EY 01769-01 and a Senior Research Fellowship by the National Retinitis Pigmentosa Foundation.

REFERENCES

Barnett, K. C. (1962) Hereditary retinal atrophy in the poodle. *Vet. Rec.* 74:672.

Bernstein, M. H. (1961) Functional architecture of the retinal epithelium, in "The Structure of the Eye" (G. K. Smelser, ed.) pp. 139-150, Academic Press, New York.

Bernstein, M. H., and Pease, D. C. (1959) Electron microscopy of the tapelucidum of the cat. *J. Biophys. Biochem. Cytol.* 5: 35-39.

Bok, D., and Hall, M. O. (1971) The role of the pigment epithelium in the etiology of inherited retinal dystrophy in the rat. *J. Cell Biol.* 49:664.

Bourne, M. C., Campbell, D. A., and Tansley, K. (1938) Hereditary degeneration of the rat retina. *Brit. J. Ophthal.* 22:613.

Bourne, M. C., and Gruneberg, H. (1939) Degeneration of the retina and cataract. A new recessive gene in the rat (*Rattus norvegicus*). *J. Hered.* 30:131.

Bruckner, R. (1951) Spaltlampenmikroskopie und ophthalmoskopie am auge von Ratte and Maus. *Doc. Ophthal.* 5-6:452.

Cogan, D. G. (1950) Symposium: Primary chorioretinal aberrations with night blindness - Pathology, 1949–1950. *Trans. Amer. Acad. Ophthal. Otolaryn.* 54:629.

Cogan, D. G. (1962) Retinal architecture and pathophysiology. The Sanford R. Gifford Lecture. *Amer. J. Ophthal.* 54:347.

Cohen, A. I. (1960) The ultrastructure of the rods of the mouse retina. *Amer. J. Anat.* 107:23.

Cohen, A. I. (1961) The fine structure of the extrafoveal receptors of the Rhesus monkey. *Exp. Eye Res.* 1:128.

Cohen, A. I. (1963) Vertebrate retinal cells and their organization. *Biol. Rev.* 38:427.

Cohrs, P. (1933) Vererbbare agenesie und hypoplasie der neuroepithelschicht der retina bei albinotischen mausen. *Arch. Augenheilk.* 107:489.

Dowling, J. E. (1967) Visual adaptation: its mechanism. *Science* 157:583.

Dowling, J. E., and Gibbons, I. R. (1962) The fine structure of the pigment epithelium in the albino rat. *J. Cell Biol.* 14:459.

Dowling, J. E., and Sidman, R. L. (1962) Inherited retinal dystrophy in the rat. *J. Cell Biol.* 14:73.

Dubin, M. W. (1970) The inner plexiform layer of the vertebrate retina, a quantitative and comparative electron microscopic analysis. *J. Comp. Neurol.* 140:479.

Gibbons, I. R., and Grimstone, A. V. (1960) On flagellar structure in certain flagella. *J. Biophys. Biochem. Cytol.* 4:697.

Green, D. G. (1971) Light adaptation in the rat retina: evidence for two receptor mechanisms. *Science* 174:598.

Herron, W. L., Riegel, B. W., Myers, O. E., and Rubin, M. L. (1969) Retinal dystrophy in the rat -- a pigment epithelial disease. *Invest. Ophthal.* 8:595.

Hogan, M. J., Alvarado, J. A., and Weddell, J. E. (1971) "Histology of the Human Eye," W. B. Saunders, Philadelphia.

Hopkins, A. E. (1927) Vision in mice with "rodless retina." *Z. Bergl. Physiol.* 6:345.

Karli, P. (1952) Retines sans cellules visuelles. Recherches morphologiques, physiologiques et physiopathologiques chez les Rongeurs. *Arch. Anat. Histol. Embryol.* 35:1.

Keeler, C. N. (1924) The inheritance of a retinal abnormality in white mice. *Proc. Nat. Acad. Sci. (USA)* 10:329.

Kolb, H., and Gouras, P. (1974) Electron microscopic observation of human retinitis pigmentosa, dominant inherited. *Invest. Ophthal.* 13:487.

Kuwabara, T., and Cogan, D. G. (1960) Tetrazolium studies on the retina. III. Activity of metabolic intermediates and miscellaneous substrates. *J. Histochem. Cytochem.* 8:214-224.

Kuwabara, T., and Cogan, D. G. (1961) Retinal glycogen. *Arch. Ophthal.* 66:680.

Kuwabara, T., and Gorn, R. A. (1968) Retinal damage by visible light. An electron microscopic study. *Arch. Ophthal.* 79:69.

Ladman, A. J. (1958) The fine structure of the rod bipolar synapse in the retina of the albino rat. *J. Biophys. Biochem. Cytol.* 4:459.

Lai, Y. L., Jacoby, R. O., Jonas, A. M., and Papermaster, D. S. (1975) A new form of hereditary retinal degeneration in Wag/Rij rats. *Invest. Ophthal.* 14:62.

LaVail, M. M., Sidman, R. L. and O'Neil, D. (1972) Photoreceptor-pigment epithelial cell relationships in rats with inherited retinal degeneration. Radioautographic and electron microscope evidence for a dual source of extra lamellar material. *J. Cell Biol.* 53:185.

LaVail, M. M., and Sidman, R. L. (1974) C57BL/6J mice with inherited retinal degeneration. *Arch. Ophthal.* 91:394.

Leure-Dupress, A. E. (1974) Observations on the synaptic organization of the retina of the albino rat. A light and electron microscopic study. *J. Comp. Neurol.* 153:149.

Lucas, D. R. (1954) Retinal dystrophy in Irish setter. *J. Exp. Zool.* 126:537.

Lucas, D. R., Attfield, M. and Davey, J. B. (1955) Retinal dystrophy in the rat. *J. Pathol. Bacteriol.* 70:469.

Menner, E. (1928) Utersuchungen uber die retina mit besonderer Berucksichtigung der ausseren Kornerschicht. Ein Beitrag zur duplizitatstheorie. *Z. vergl. Physiol.* viii:761.

Noell, W. K., Walker, V. S., Kang, B. S., and Berman, S. (1966) Retinal damage by light in rats. *Invest. Ophthal.* 5:450.

O'Steen, W. K. (1970) Retinal and optic nerve serotonin and retinal degeneration as influenced by photoperiod. *Exp. Neurol.* 27:194.

O'Steen, W. K., and Anderson, K. V. (1971) Photically-evoked responses in the visual system of rats exposed to continuous light. *Exp. Neurol.* 30:525.

O'Steen, W. K., and Anderson, K. V. (1972) Photoreceptor degeneration after exposure of rats to incandescent illumination. *Z. Zellf.* 127:306.

Parry, H. B. (1953) Degenerations of the dog retina. II. Generalized progressive atrophy of hereditary origin. *Brit. J. Ophthal.* 37:487.

Reynolds, E. S. (1963) The use of lead citrate at high pH as an electron-opaque stain in electron microscopy. *J. Cell Biol.* 17:208.

Richardson, K. G., Jarett, L., and Finke, E. H. (1960) Embedding in epoxy resins for ultrathin sectioning in electron microscopy. *Stain Tech.* 35:313.

Sidman, R. L. (1958) Histochemical studies on photoreceptor cells. *Ann. N. Y. Acad. Sci.* 74:182.

Sjostrand, F. S. (1960) Electron microscopy of myeline and of nerve cells and tissue, in "Modern Scientific Aspects of Neurology" (J. N. Cumings, ed.) p. 118, Arnold, Ltd., London.

Sorsby, A., Koller, P. C., Attfield, M., Davey, J. B. and Lucas, D. R. (1954) Retinal dystrophy in the mouse: histological and genetic aspect. *J. Exp. Zool.* 125:171.

Sosula, L., and Glow, P. H. (1970) A quantitative ultrastructural study of the inner plexiform layer of the rat retina. *J. Comp. Neurol.* 140:439.

Spurr, A. R. (1969) A low-viscosity epoxy resin embedding medium for electron microscopy. *J. Ultrastruc. Res.* 26:31.

Tansley, K. (1951)   Hereditary   degeneration of the   mouse retina. *Brit. J. Ophthal.* 35:573.

Verhoeff, F. H. (1931)   Microscopic observations in a case of reti- nitis pigmentosa. *Arch. Ophthal.* 5:392.

Walls, G. L. (1936)   The   visual   cells   of the   white   rat. *Comp. Psychol.* 18:364.

Wislocki, G. B., and   Ladman, A. J. (1955)   The   demonstration of a blood-ocular   barrier   in the albino rat by means of the intra- vitam deposition of silver. *J. Biophys. Biochem. Cytol.* 1:501.

Yamada, E., Tokuyasu, K., and   Iwaki, S. (1958)   The fine structure of retina   studied with the electron microscope. II.   Pigment epithelium and   capillaries of the   choriocapillary layer. *J. Electronmicros.* 42:5.

EXPLANATION OF ABBREVIATIONS IN FIGURES

A	apical microvilli	L	lysosome
C	cone cell	Lf	lipofuscin granules
do	disintegrated outer segments	N	mitochondria
D	degenerated cell	ON	outer nuclear layer
E	basal infoldings	OS	outer segment
G	cytoplasmic inclusion	P	pigment epithelium
IN	inner nuclear layer	cp	cone pedicle
IS	inner segment	s	rod spherule

THE DYSTROPHIC RAT AS A MODEL FOR CLINICAL RESEARCH

Warren L. Herron, Jr.

Department of Ophthalmology
University of Florida
Gainesville, Florida 32601

The pathophysiology of retinal dystrophy in the rat may be entirely unrelated to any human disease. A parallel pathophysiology to the rat has not been encountered in other reported animal dystrophies. It is also simplistic to assume that one pathological mechanism can be expected to account for all human retinal dystrophies.

However, the rat shares many similar findings with retinal dystrophy in man. These similar findings include genetic transmission. Both species show a progressive deterioration in the ERG which finally becomes extinguished (Dowling and Sidman, 1962). The ophthalmoscopic appearance of the rat (Herron *et al*., 1974) is quite similar to that of man. It must be remembered that the pigmentary changes are secondary in the rat and that the progressive retinal vascular alteration and pallor of the disc are also secondary (Fig. 1). It is quite likely that the retinal pigmentary findings in man, as well as the disc and vascular changes, are similarly induced. Some rats, like man, show a distinct border between thinned degenerated retina with prominent pigmentary change and the thicker, still functioning retinal areas. Finally, end stage histology in man and rat are similar.

The rat is currently the only dystrophic model where the pathophysiologic course is understood. Alteration of the normal rod photoreceptor outer segment renewal and pigment epithelial phagocytosis process is the basic cause of retinal dystrophy in the rat. [In the normal state there is continual renewal of rod outer segment material with the distal lamellae being phagocytized by the pigment epithelium (Young, 1967; Young and Bok, 1969).] The dystrophic rat shows an absolute inability of the pigment epithelial cells to phagocytize its rod outer segment material (Herron *et al*., 1969, 1971; Bok and Hall, 1971; LaVail *et al*., 1972) (Fig.

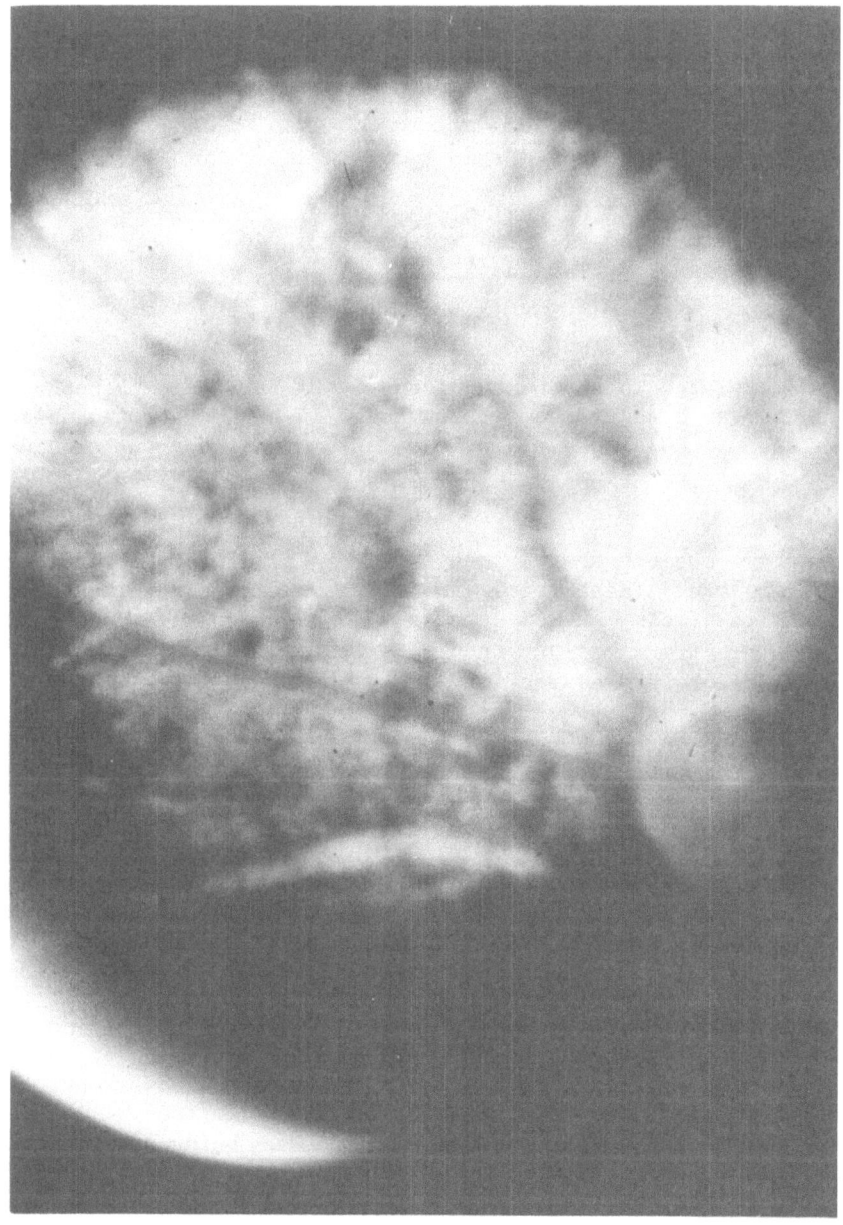

FIGURE 1. Dystrophic pigmented rat fundus, age 20 weeks. The retina is very thin and shows clumped pigment, markedly narrowed vessels and paleness of the optic disc.

2). Its pigment epithelial cells can phagocytize latex spheres
(Fig. 3),   thorotrast (Fig. 4),   and india ink (Fig. 5), but apparently not rod outer segments (Herron, 1972; Brennan and Herron,
1973; Bok and Lloyd, 1973). However, rod outer segments from
dystrophic rats can be phagocytized by normal rat pigment epithelial cells *in vitro* (Brennan and Herron, 1973).

     The key problem appears to be at the membrane level.   In
normal rats, rod outer segment material has been shown to be phago-
cytizable by the pigment epithelium only after light exposure and a
period of time has occurred (Herron and Riegel, 1974a). Until this
duration of time-light has occurred, the pigment epithelium benign-
ly sits adjacent to the outer segment material and does not engulf
it. This is well illustrated in severe vitamin A deficiency, in
which rod outer segment material stays up to five times longer
adjacent to the pigment epithelial processes, but is not removed
until the normal ten day interval has elapsed (Herron and Riegel,
1974a). These findings in vitamin A deficiency serve to help
explain the documented findings by Dowling and Sidman (1962), that
light deprivation in the dystrophic animals distinctly slows the
degeneration, as well as the recent report that lack of pigmentation increases the speed of retinal degeneration, as shown by
LaVail (LaVail and Battelle, 1975). Thus, the induced variations
in the rate of retinal degeneration in the dystrophic rat, whether
caused by light (Dowling and Sidman, 1962; Young, 1967), lack of
absorption of light (LaVail and Battelle, 1975), temperature variation (Young, 1967), and/or increased metabolic rate can all be
explained as affecting the rate of the breakdown of rod outer segment material in a system where phagocytosis of the disrupted rod
outer segment lamellae does not take place. In the dystrophic rat,
there is no equilibrium between rod outer segment production and
pigment epithelial removal.

     The slower time course in human dystrophy could be explained
by a relative defect in rod outer segment removal. An alternate
explanation could be that the cones, which do not show outer segment lamellar production in their normal state (Young, 1971), help
retinal survival by not contributing to the buildup of debris.
This would help explain the initial mid-peripheral field loss in
human dystrophy, because this is the area of highest rod concentration. As more time elapses, the far periphery, where cells are
less closely spaced, ceases to function. Finally, only after many
years, and frequently not within a lifetime, is the central foveal
all-cone area destroyed.

     In summary, therapeutic approaches based on the dystrophic
rat model are most logically aimed at restoring the normal rod
outer segment pigment epithelial interrelationships. Simply, one
needs to make the pigment epithelium eat rod outer segment material. If this cannot be accomplished, or until it can be done,

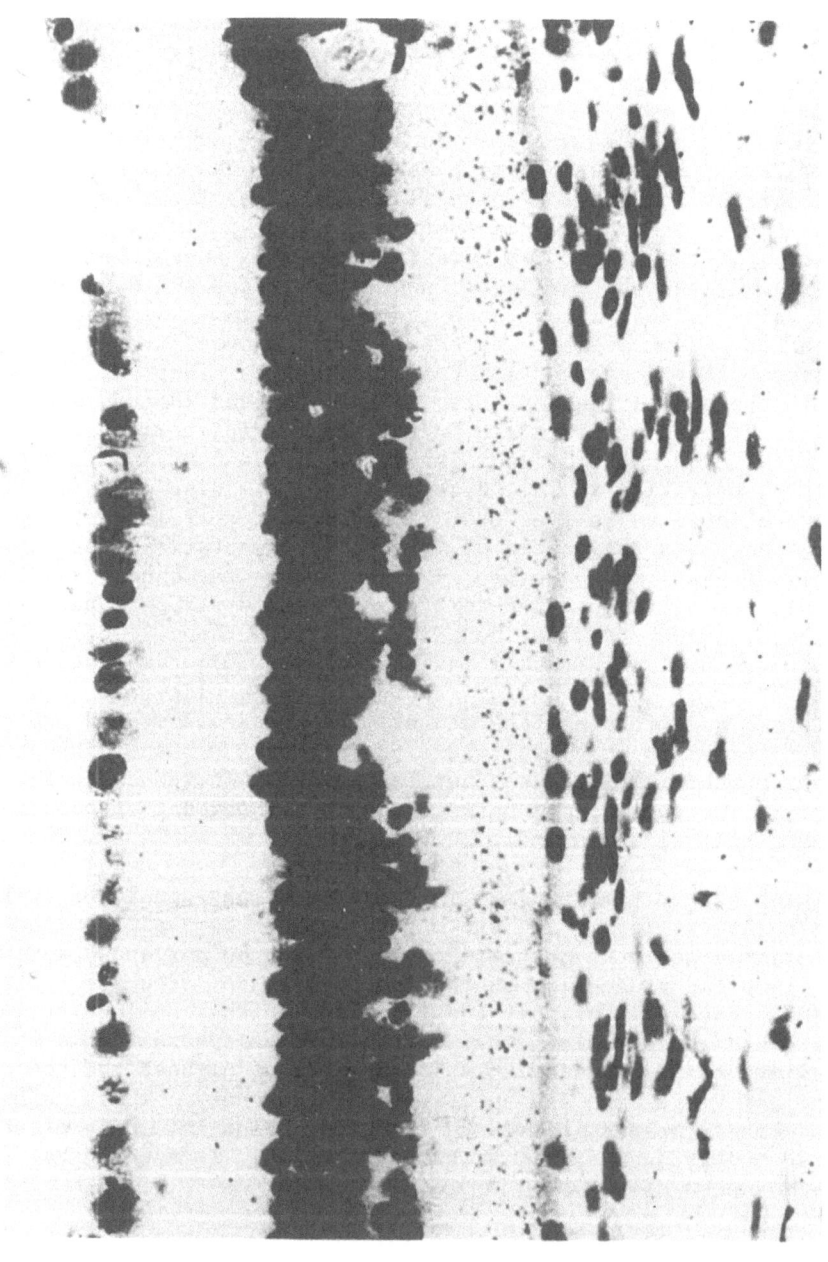

FIGURE 2. Autoradiograph of the retina of a dystrophic rat. Choroid and pigment epithelium are to the top of the photograph and inner retinal layers are below. The animal was injected at 10 days of age with tritiated amino acid. The band of labeled rod outer segment material has persisted for 120 days from the time of injection adjacent to the pigment epithelium. It has not been phagocytized by the pigment epithelium. More recently produced outer segment material and most of the photoreceptor cell nuclei have degenerated and been removed, presumably through the inner retina.

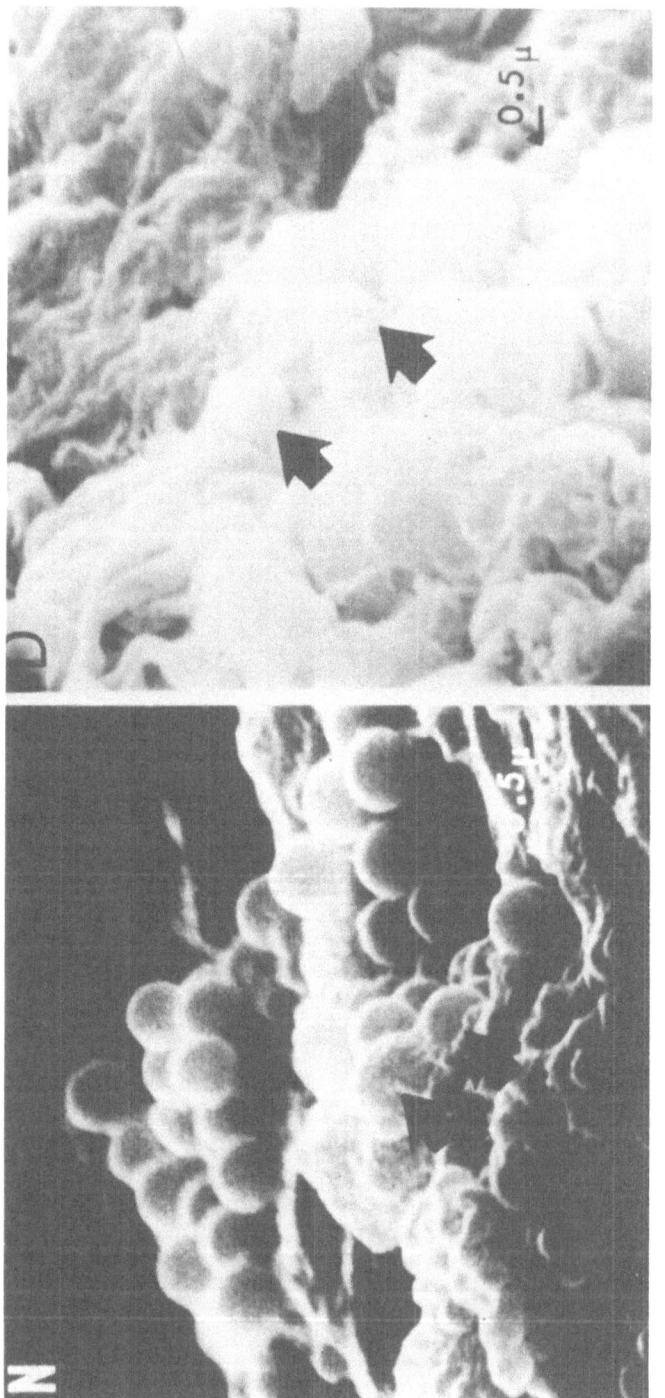

FIGURE 3. Scanning electron microscope (EM) photo of latex spheres showing phagocytosis by normal (N) and dystrophic (D) rat pigment epithelium in whole mount.

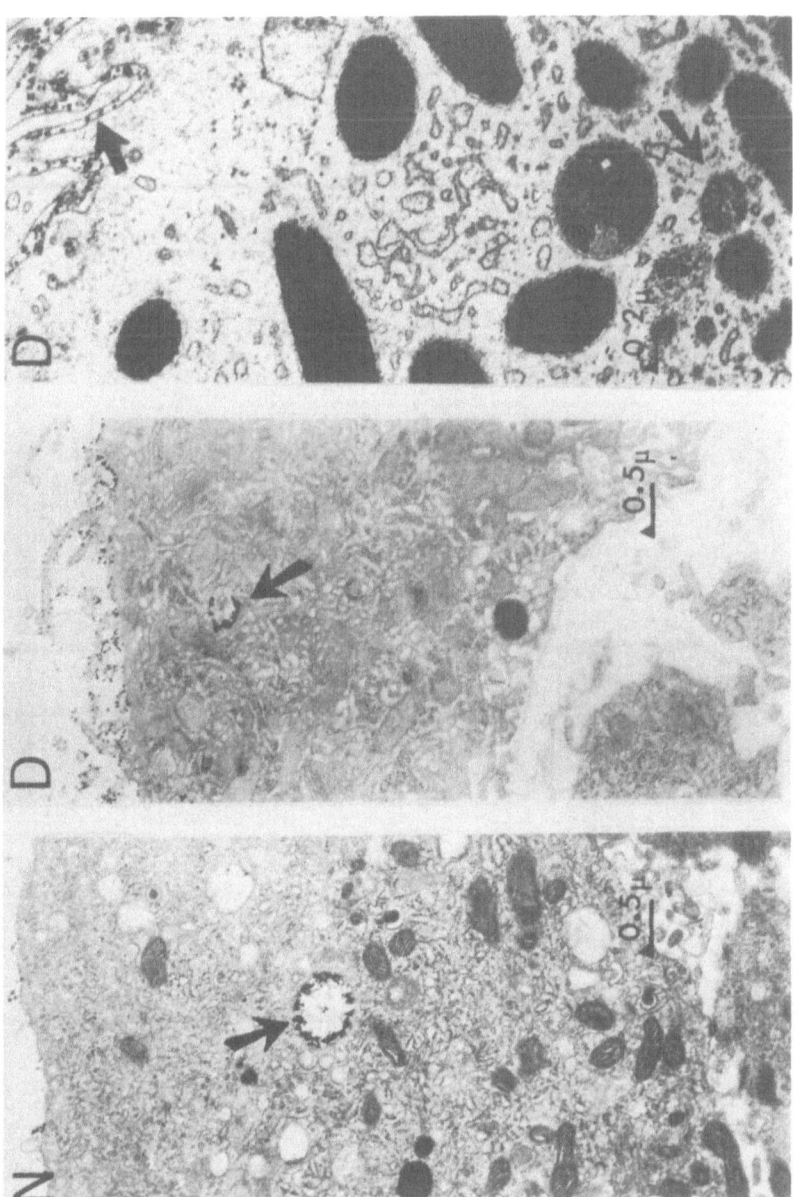

FIGURE 4. Transmission EM photo of normal (N) and dystrophic (D) pigment epithelium showing phagocytosis of thorotrast by each. Also note accumulation of thorotrast at pigment epithelial processes in dystrophic pigment epithelial cell at right. Cells were whole mount preparations.

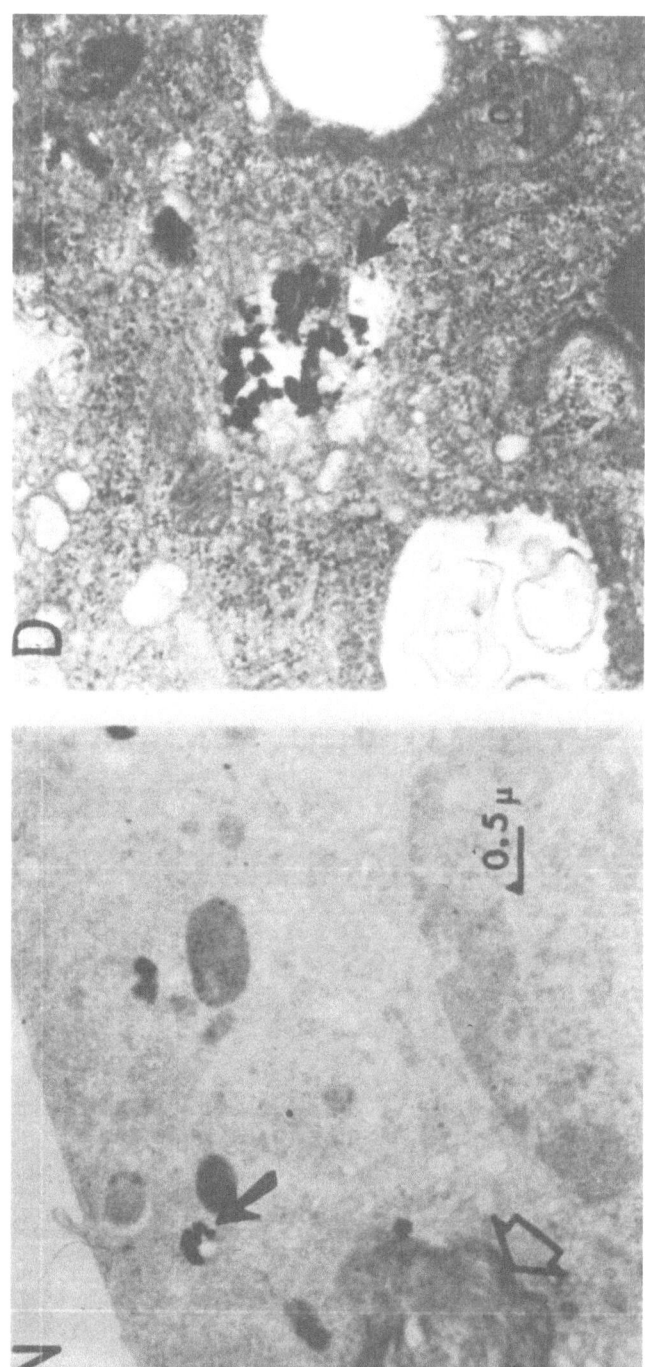

FIGURE 5. Transmission EM photo of normal (N) and dystrophic (D) pigment epithelium showing phagocytosis of india ink. Cells were from whole mount preparations.

additional therapeutic approaches are available for normalizing this basic rod outer segment production-pigment epithelium removal equilibrium: (1) altering the production rate of rod outer segment material; (2) altering the quantity of rod outer segment material; (3) altering the breakdown of rod outer segment material.

1. The production rate of rod outer segment material can be decreased by vitamin A deficiency (Herron and Riegel, 1974a) (Fig. 6). As vitamin A deficiency increases, the rate of rod outer segment production decreases. Thus, less and less rod outer segment material needs to be removed by the pigment epithelium. Low levels of vitamin A deficiency can significantly decrease the rod outer segment lamellar production.

2. Vitamin A deficiency can result in permanent rod photo-receptor death (Herron and Riegel, 1974b). As more and more rods are killed by vitamin A deficiency, less and less rod outer segment material will be produced when the deficient state is terminated. Thus, vitamin A deficiency can permanently alter the amount of rod outer segment material subsequently produced by the retina (Fig. 7).

An additional benefit of vitamin A deficiency is that it protects the photoreceptor cells from light damage, as Noell and co-workers have so beautifully shown (Noell *et al.*, 1971). This benefit of vitamin A deficiency could work for cones as well as rods, and may be the most compelling reason to even consider vitamin A deficiency in humans.

If vitamin A deficiency therapy is to be considered to alter the quantity of rod outer segment material, it must obviously be done before all of the rods are destroyed. Thus, young patients with near normal fields and dark adaptation would be the most likely candidates. The better the ERG, the more likely we are to get useful data. The value of retinoic acid in protecting from the dangers of vitamin A deficiency needs to be carefully evaluated prior to use on humans. In our laboratory, rats on a retinoic acid and vitamin A test diet with additional vitamin supplements did poorly. [John Dowling did not have trouble with rats on vitamin A test diet and retinoic acid. They did as well as the non-deficient animals. Our animals on test diet did not gain weight or have shiny coats in any way comparable to those on normal laboratory diet, though they did not die. A possible explanation for this discrepancy is that we fed our animals commercially prepared vitamin A test diet, with frequently purchased new small batches. Dr. Dowling prepared his test diet himself and, therefore, was quite certain of its ingredients and freshness. There is, therefore, the possibility that the test diet is the cause of the poor growth of our experimental animals, and not the retinoic acid.] In the Long Evans rats on vitamin A deficiency with retinoic acid,

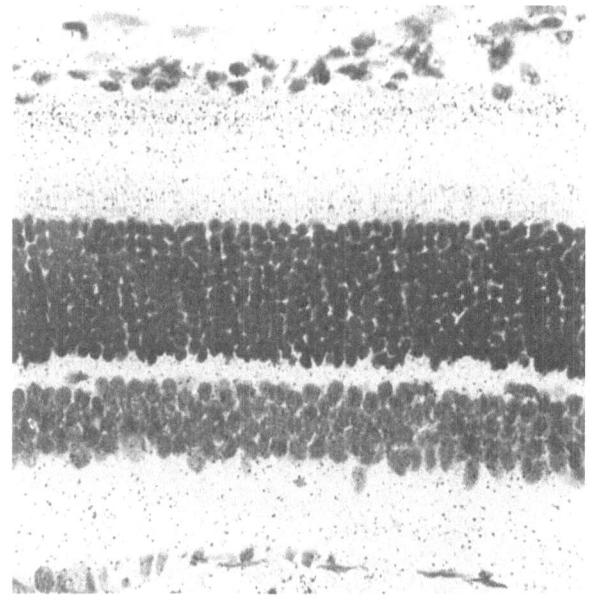

FIGURE 6.1

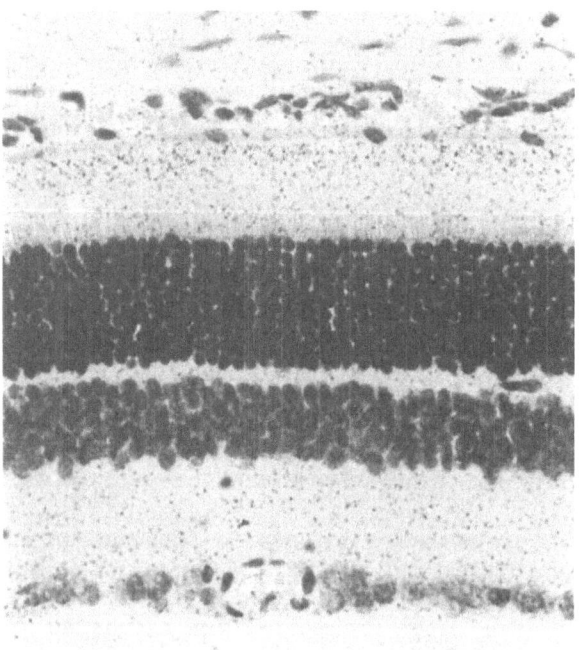

FIGURE 6.2

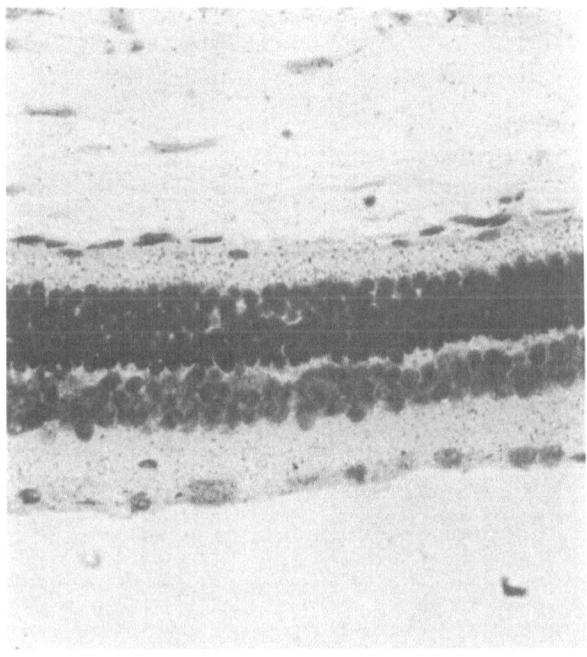

FIGURE 6.3

FIGURE 6. Each micrograph at 40X shows autoradiograph 10 days after injection of tritiated methionine. Each micrograph shows the radiolabel in the distal outer segment material near the pigment epithelium. Therefore, the turnover of any outer segment lamellae from production to phagocytosis takes the same time-light interval (10 days). Since the more deficient animals have a thinner layer of rod outer segments, it is apparent that they have a slower production rate of rod outer segment lamellae and also that these more slowly produced lamellae are adjacent to the pigment epithelium for a longer time interval before phagocytic removal. The thickness of the layer of rods decreases as the vitamin A deficiency increases. [6.1] Control rat with normal ERG. [6.2] Vitamin A deficient, 85 days on diet and ERG 4 log units deficient. [6.3] Vitamin A deficient, 111 days on diet and ERG more than 6 log units deficient.

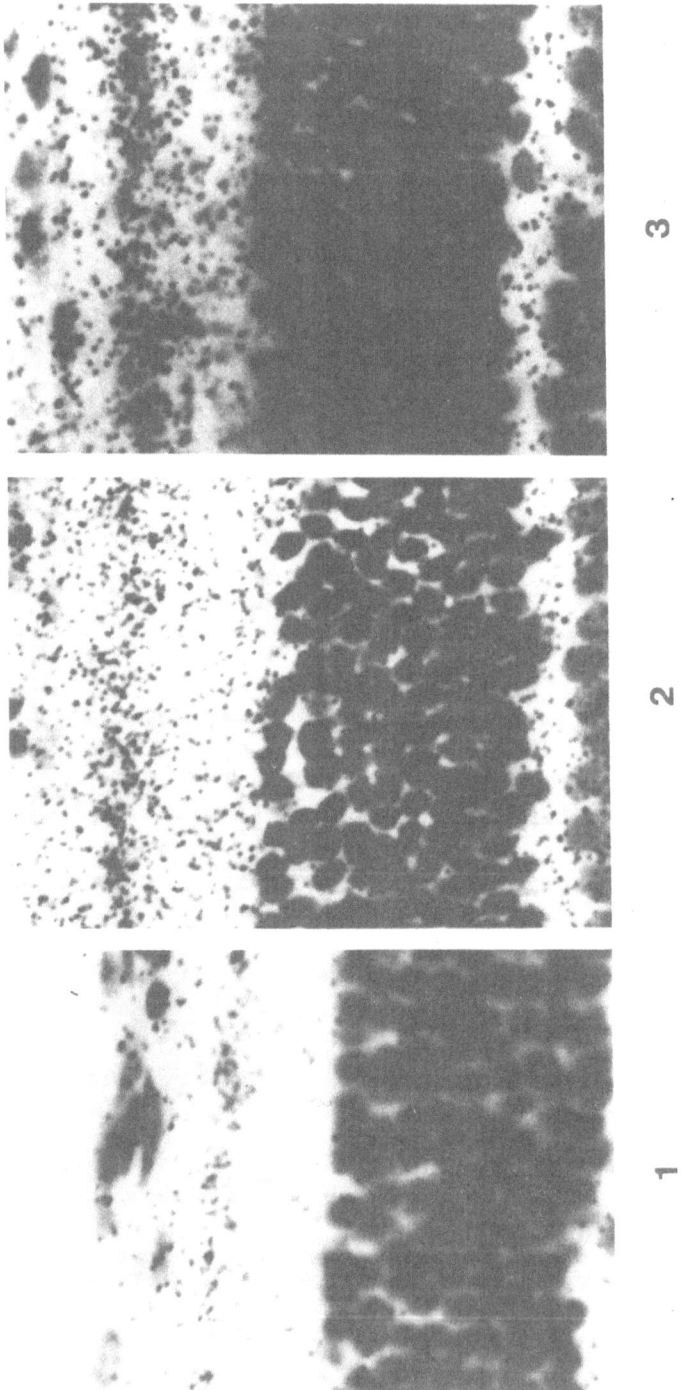

FIGURE 7. [7.1] Vitamin A deficient animal "B" at five days after injection of radiolabel 10 μCi per gram of NET – 153 L-phenylalanine^{3}H-G (0.183 mg = 5 μCi) and 10 μCi per gram of NET – 135 A L-leucine 4.5 ^{3}H (0.017 mg = 5 μCi). [7.2] Other eye of animal "B" at two weeks and five days from administration of 10,000 μ aqueous vitamin A (Aquasol) intraperitoneally and five days after identical dosage of tracer at 10 μCi per gram of both tracers. [7.3] Control animal at five days after injection of 10 μCi per gram of both tracers.

NOTE: All animals show label midway in the layer of rods. Radio label density increases progressively from one to three. Thickness of the layer of rods increases significantly from one to three.

cataracts were frequently encountered after long periods. Thus, at this time we do not feel that severe levels of vitamin A deficiency on human patients can be justified on merely theoretical grounds. Carefully monitored low levels of deficiency might give useful information without undue risk. However, blood vitamin A levels and general health must be very carefully monitored and childbearing avoided.

3. A third approach at altering the rod outer segment production-pigment epithelium removal equilibrium entails altering the break-down of rod outer segment material. This should be responsive to decreasing metabolic rate, decreasing temperature, and light restriction. Light restriction is quite popular, as has been already noted. It has been shown to prolong the ERG in the dystrophic rat, and so it is a proven rat technique. Perhaps it works because decreasing light slows the breakdown and new production of rod outer segment material in the dystrophic rat. Perhaps it is effective because, in so doing, the normal flow of nutrition between the choriocapillaris and the photoreceptor outer segments is not interrupted by the old rod outer segment debris and pigment epithelial processes and swirls. [The buildup of old rod outer segment debris is not comparable to a similar displacement from the choriocapillaris by, for example, pigment epithelial cells, as the cells are living with active transport mechanisms and the debris is extracellular degeneration products.]

There is theoretical and experimental reason to avoid intermittent episodes of total light restriction and sporadic light exposure with the subsequent rapid breakdown of rod outer segment material (Noell et al., 1971; Kuwabara and Gorn, 1968). Experiments should be tailored to avoid this, if possible. Again, if the dystrophic rat is the model used for human dystrophy, one would want to institute therapy when viable rods are still present. However, in any retina that is nutritionally limited, even with only cones remaining, light deprivation could help the metabolically stressed system survive.

In selecting a lens for these purposes, I would consider dark red the ideal color. It would allow little stimulation of the rhodopsin as it is well beyond the λ max, and if it is of longer wavelength than seen in a protanopic spectral sensitivity curve, it would spare the range of the other "non-red" cones. Patient acceptance will determine what lenses can be used.

In the very young, light deprivation can most easily be done with miotics. If phospholine iodide can be used for accommodative esotropes, miotics are probably not too hazardous to be considered for patients with retinal dystrophies.

Only well designed, carefully controlled experiments carried out over many years will enable us to get useful data in our attempts to help control human retinal dystrophies.

In the meantime, it is hoped that someone will determine a way to correct the basic biochemical defects so the stopgap therapies we are considering can be forgotten.

REFERENCES

Bok, D., and Hall, M. O. (1971) The role of the pigment epithelium in the etiology of inherited retinal dystrophy in the rat. *J. Cell. Biol.* 49:664.

Bok, D., and Lloyd, M. (1973) E/M histochemical studies on the pigmented epithelium of dystrophic rat retinas. Annual meeting of the Association for Research in Vision and Ophthalmology, Sarasota, Florida, Abstract # 11, p. 7.

Brennan, F. E., and Herron, W. L., Jr. (1973) Comparison of phagocytosis by normal and dystrophic rat retinal pigment epithelium. Annual meeting of the Association for Research in Vision and Ophthalmology, Sarasota, Florida, Abstract #4, p. 16.

Dowling, J. E., and Sidman, R. L. (1962) Inherited retinal dystrophy in the rat. *J. Cell. Biol.* 14:73.

Herron, W. L., Jr. (1972) Normal photoreceptor and pigment epithelium interrelationships and characteristics which pertain to inherited retinal dystrophy. Annual meeting of the Association for Research in Vision and Ophthalmology, Sarasota, Fla.

Herron, W. L., Jr., and Riegel, B. W. (1974a) Production rate and removal of rod outer segment material in vitamin A deficiency. *Invest. Ophthal.* 13:46.

Herron, W. L., Jr., and Riegel, B. W. (1974b) Vitamin A deficiency induced "rod thinning" to permanently decrease the production of rod outer segment material. *Invest. Ophthal.* 13:54.

Herron, W. L., Jr., Riegel, B. W., Myers, O. E., and Rubin, M. L. (1969) Retinal dystrophy in the rat -- a pigment epithelial disease. *Invest. Ophthal.* 8:595.

Herron, W. L., Jr., Riegel, B. W., and Rubin, M. L. (1971) Outer segment production and removal in the degenerating retina of the dystrophic rat. *Invest. Ophthal.* 10:54.

Herron, W. L., Jr., Riegel, B. W., Brennan, F. E., and Rubin, M. L. (1974) Retinal dystrophy in the pigmented rat. *Invest. Ophthal.* 13:87.

Kuwabara, T., and Gorn, R. A. (1968) Retinal damage by visible light: an electron microscopic study. *Arch. Ophthal.* 79:69.

LaVail, M. M., and Battelle, B.-A. (1975) Influence of eye pigmentation and light deprivation on inherited retinal dystrophy in the rat. *Exp. Eye Res.* 21:167.

LaVail, M. M., Sidman, R. L., and O'Neil, D. (1972) Photoreceptor-pigment epithelial cell relationships in rats with inherited retinal degeneration: radioautographic and electron microscopic evidence for a dual source of extra lamellar material. *J. Cell. Biol.* 53:185.

Noell, W. K., Delmelle, M. C., and Albrecht, R. (1971) Vitamin A deficiency effect on retina: dependence on light. *Science* 17:72.

Young, R. W. (1967) The renewal of photoreceptor cell outer segments. *J. Cell. Biol.* 33:61.

Young, R. W. (1971) The renewal of rod and cone outer segments in the rhesus monkey. *J. Cell. Biol.* 49:303.

Young, R. W., and Bok, D. (1969) Participation of the retinal pigment epithelium in the rod outer segment renewal process. *J. Cell. Biol.* 42:392.

EXPERIMENTAL CHIMERAS: A NEW APPROACH TO THE STUDY OF INHERITED

RETINAL DEGENERATION IN LABORATORY ANIMALS

Matthew M. LaVail and Richard J. Mullen

Department of Neuropathology, Harvard Medical School
Department of Neuroscience, Children's Hospital Medical
    School
Boston, Massachusetts   02115

INTRODUCTION

Few details are known about cytopathological events in the early stages of retinitis pigmentosa (RP) or in any of the inherited retinal degenerations in man. For this reason, there has been considerable interest in laboratory animals which share with the human retinal diseases the selective and progressive hereditary degeneration of photoreceptors. Several breeds of dogs (see review in Aguirre and Rubin, 1976), several strains of rats (see review in LaVail, 1976), and mice with several specific mutations (see review in LaVail and Sidman, 1974; Mullen and LaVail, 1975) are known to have inherited retinal degenerations. The most widely studied have been retinal degeneration in the mouse (gene symbol rd) and retinal dystrophy in the rat (gene symbol rdy). Both are recessively inherited disorders and have been the object of numerous morphologic, biochemical, electrophysiologic, genetic and behavioral studies.

The discovery of a disorder in the pigment epithelium in RCS rats with inherited retinal dystrophy has directed the attention of investigators in vision research to one of the basic problems in dealing with cell degenerations in the central nervous system, that of defining the precise cellular localization of a genetic defect. In RCS rats the pigment epithelial cells fail to phagocytize rod outer segment discs which leads to an accumulation of outer segment membranes (Herron *et al.*, 1969; Bok and Hall, 1971; LaVail and Battelle, 1975). On the one hand, it has been suggested that this accumulation results from a primary pigment epithelial cell defect (Herron *et al.*, 1969). On the other hand, it has been proposed

that an abnormality in the rod outer segments leads to secondary
involvement of the pigment epithelium (Burden *et al.*, 1971).
Indeed, until shown otherwise, it can also be argued that the pigment epithelium or photoreceptor cells may be the target of a
systemic or circulating factor. This example in the RCS rat illu-
strates the fact that any inherited photoreceptor degeneration may
result not only from a primary genetic defect in the photoreceptor
cell, but also from defects in the pigment epithelial cell, other
cells in the neural retina, or even from factors extrinsic to the
eye.

We have been studying this problem in mice with retinal
degeneration and in rats with retinal dystrophy by the use of
experimental chimeras (LaVail and Mullen, 1976; Mullen and LaVail,
1976). Chimeras are produced that contain mixtures of genetically
mutant and genetically normal cells. By using different pigmentation genotypes, mutant and normal pigment epithelial cells can be
identified on the basis of pigmentation, and the interaction of
both types of cells with the adjacent neural retina can then be
analyzed by morphological methods. In this chapter, we will first
describe the production of chimeras and general methods of analyz-
ing chimeric retinas, review the findings thus far obtained with
mouse chimeras and rat chimeras, and finally discuss some of the
limitations and future applications of experimental chimeras in
vision research.

DESCRIPTION AND PRODUCTION OF EXPERIMENTAL CHIMERAS

"Chimeras" are mythological fire-breathing monsters, commonly
represented with a lion's head, a goat's body and a serpent's tail.
A more modern, biological definition of a chimera is an organism
composed of tissues containing two or more genetically distinct
cell classes derived from two embryos. In the early 1960's, Tarkowski (1961) and Mintz (1962, 1965) developed the technique of
fusing mouse embryos from different strains and produced experimental mouse chimeras that displayed mosaicism in a variety of organ
systems. In the ensuing years, mouse chimeras have been used as a
tool for studying many developmental problems (see review by Mintz,
1974). The experimental mouse chimeras are also called fusion chimeras, allophenic mice, tetraparental mice or mosaic mice. (The
various tissues in these mice are mosaics of genetically different
cells; however, reference to an organism as a mosaic generally
implies development from a single zygote, not from two as in the
case of the chimeric mice.)

The details of the procedure we use for producing chimeric
mice have been described by Mullen and Whitten (1971). It consists
of flushing eight-cell embryos from the oviducts on day 2.5 (day of
mating - day 0), removing the zona pellucida with pronase and

allowing the embryos of two different genotypes to aggregate over-
night in culture. The chimeric blastocysts are then surgically
transplanted into the uteri of pregnant or pseudopregnant females
for the remainder of gestation. The procedure is the same for rat
chimeras except the embryos are collected on day 3.5. The chimeric
animals are identified usually by mosaicism of coat color (Fig. 1)
and sometimes by eye pigmentation (Figs. 2, 3), assuming that
embryos with different pigmentation genotypes were used. The symbol "↔" (Mintz, 1964) is conventionally used to indicate chimeras
derived from two embryos of different genotypes or strains (e.g.,
rd/rd ↔ +/+ or C3H ↔ C57BL/6J).

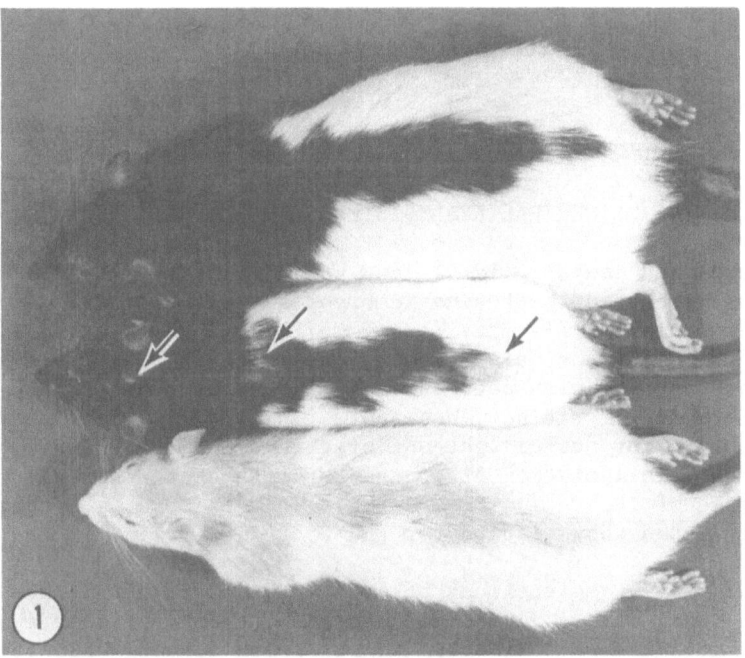

FIGURE 1. Example of a rat chimera (middle) and its two parental
    strain phenotypes. Retinal dystrophic RCS rats are tan-hooded
    (below). Fischer X RCS F_1 hybrid rats (above) are black-
    hooded and are +/rdy at the retinal dystrophy locus. In the
    RCS ↔ (Fischer X RCS)F_1 chimera (middle), patches of tan
    (RCS) pigmentation are indicated by arrows on the head and in
    the otherwise black hood.

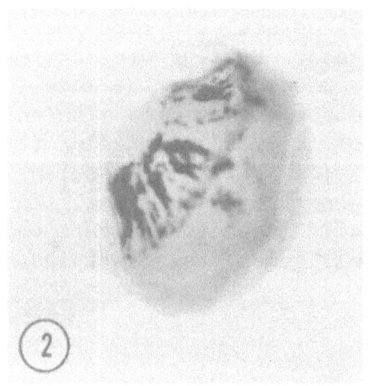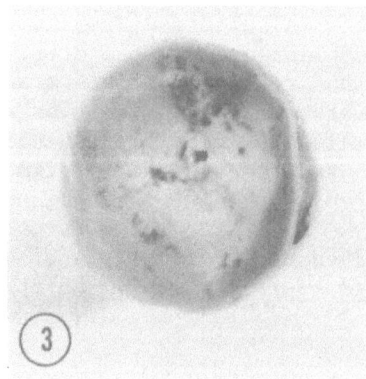

FIGURES 2, 3. Lateral (Fig. 2) and posterior (Fig. 3) views of an
eye from an albino ↔ pigmented mouse chimera demonstrating
pigmentation mosaicism.

GENERAL ANALYSIS OF CHIMERIC RETINAS

Mintz and Sanyal (1970) and Wegmann *et al.* (1971) found in
chimeras produced by fusing embryos of C3H (rd/rd) mice with
those of normal (+/+) mice (e.g., C57BL/10), that the retinas displayed a patchy retinal degeneration. Patches of normal retina
were interspersed with patches lacking photoreceptors, and regions
of "intermediate" retina (Wegmann *et al.*, 1971) with several rows
of photoreceptor nuclei instead of the normal 8-10 rows were present either in isolation or at the borders of the normal patches.
An example of the retina from a C3H ↔ B10 chimera is shown in Fig.
4. (B10 is an abbreviation for the C57BL/10 strain.)

The pigment epithelium of both C3H and C57BL/10 mice is pigmented, and so in C3H ↔ B10 chimeras, those pigment epithelial
cells that were genetically rd/rd could not be phenotypically
distinguished from those that were +/+. However, by selecting different strains of mice, one of which was albino (c/c), Mintz and
Sanyal (1970) and LaVail and Mullen (1976) were able to distinguish
the two genotypes. For example, the albino SJL strain (rd/rd c/c)
was substituted for the C3H strain, so that in SJL ↔ B10 chimeras,
pigment epithelial cells that were genotypically rd/rd could easily
be identified because they were phenotypically albino. Other
strain combinations were used such that the rd/rd pigment epithelial cells were pigmented and the +/+ cells were albino.

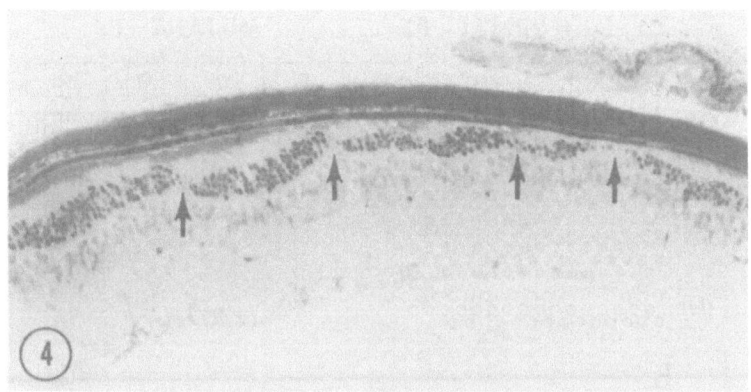

FIGURE 4. Retina from a C3H ↔ C57BL/10 mouse chimera demonstrating patches of retina with photoreceptor cells surviving
interspersed with patches lacking photoreceptors (arrows).
Mosaicism in the pigment epithelium is not evident because
both parental strains are pigmented. Epon-Araldite. One to
1.5 μm. Toluidine blue. X 175.

In the c/c rd/rd ↔ +/+ +/+ mouse chimeras, it was found that
the distribution of patches of degenerated photoreceptor cells was
independent of the genotype of the adjacent pigment epithelium.
Mintz and Sanyal (1970) and Mintz (1974) interpreted this to mean
that the developmental lineages of adjacent pigment epithelium and
photoreceptor cells are independent of one another although both
are derived from the optic vesicle. LaVail and Mullen (1976) later
pointed out that these chimeras could be used to study the cellular
localization of mutant gene expression.

The general approach to the analysis of the chimeric retinas
is illustrated in a series of different degeneration patterns in
Fig. 5. These diagrams show the degeneration pattern expected if
the mutant gene is expressed in (a) the pigment epithelial cell,
(b) the photoreceptor cell, or (c) both. If the mutant gene is
expressed only in the pigment epithelial cell and this secondarily
results in photoreceptor cell death, then photoreceptor cells
opposite mutant pigment epithelial cells should degenerate and
those opposite normal pigment epithelial cells should survive (Fig.
5a). If the mutant gene is expressed in only the photoreceptor
cell, then those photoreceptors that are genetically mutant should
degenerate, regardless of the genotype of the adjacent pigment epithelial cells (Fig. 5b). If mutant gene expression is required in

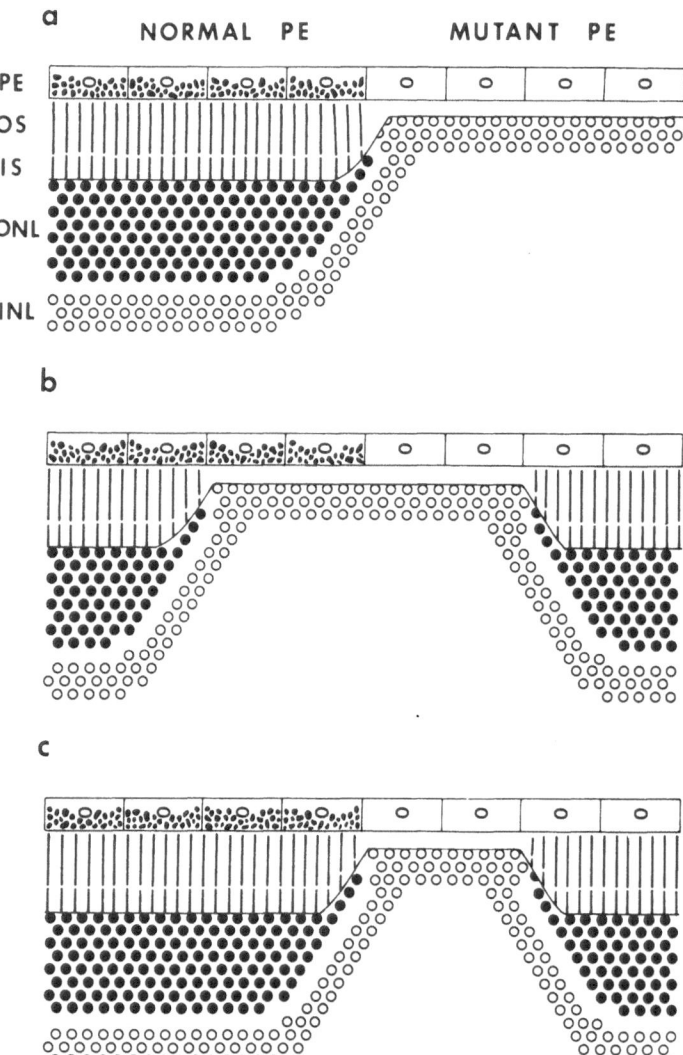

FIGURE 5. Hypothetical degeneration patterns that would be expected if photoreceptor cell death results from the mutant gene
acting in (a) the pigment epithelial cell, (b) the photoreceptor cell (or in some other cell in the neural retina, or (c)
both sites. The normal pigment epithelial cells (PE) are
drawn as pigmented and the mutant ones as albino. INL, inner
nuclear layer; IS, inner segments; ONL, outer nuclear layer;
OS, outer segments.

both cell types for photoreceptor cells to degenerate, then photo-receptor cell degeneration should be restricted to regions opposite mutant pigment epithelial cells, and those photoreceptors that are genetically normal should survive opposite mutant pigment epithe-lial cells (Fig. 5c). If photoreceptor degeneration is a result of factors extrinsic to the eye, for example, involving a circulating toxic factor, a uniform effect should exist in the chimeras with all normal, all degenerated or all intermediate retina in the two eyes of a given animal.

There are additional issues, such as pleiotropic effects of gene mutations and local interactions among cells that might modify or hinder the general chimeric analysis just described. These will be discussed after brief descriptions of the retinas of chimeric mice and rats.

OBSERVATIONS ON THE RETINAS OF CHIMERIC MICE

In retinal degeneration in the mouse, photoreceptors degen-erate and begin to disappear on about postnatal day 10, as seen by light microscopy. Few rod outer segments are ever formed. The loss of cells proceeds rapidly, and by day 20, only an incomplete row of photoreceptor nuclei remains (Figs. 6-8). Most of these will disappear in the ensuing months (LaVail and Sidman, 1974). Morphologic (Sanyal and Bal, 1973; Blanks *et al.*, 1974) and bio-chemical (Lolley, 1973; Schmidt and Lolley, 1973; Farber and Lolley, 1974) abnormalities have been found in photoreceptors before the overt degeneration of the cells. However, the important consideration for the chimeric analysis is that the eyes be taken at or near the expected end-stage of cytopathology (i.e., after 20 days of age in the mouse) in order for distinct patches of degen-erated retina to be recognizable.

In the chimeric mouse retinas examined after 20 days of age, we found normal retina adjacent to both rd/rd and +/+ pigment epi-thelial cells (Fig. 9). Similarly, we found both degenerated and intermediate retina adjacent to both genotypes of pigment epithe-lial cells (Figs. 10, 11). Further details on strain combinations,

patch distributions, outer segment renewal studies and fine structural observations are presented in LaVail and Mullen (1976).
However, the most important finding in the present context was that
the lack of correspondence of degenerated retina with rd/rd pigment
epithelium closely fits the diagram in Fig. 5b. This led us to
conclude that the pigment epithelial cell is not the primary target
of the mutant rd gene in the mouse (LaVail and Mullen, 1976).

OBSERVATIONS ON THE RETINAS OF CHIMERIC RATS

Retinal dystrophy in the rat has different cytopathologic features and time course than retinal degeneration in the mouse. In
retinal dystrophy, rod outer segments are formed, but because the
pigment epithelial cells fail to phagocytize rod outer segments
(Herron *et al.*, 1969; Bok and Hall, 1971), outer segment membranes
(debris) accumulate at the surface of the pigment epithelium.
Pyknotic photoreceptor nuclei are first seen at about day 20, and
most of the photoreceptor nuclei are missing by about day 60 in
pink-eyed animals (Figs. 12-14). Black eye pigmentation slows the
rate of photoreceptor degeneration, but most photoreceptor nuclei
are missing from pigmented retinal dystrophic rats by about day 90
(LaVail and Battelle, 1975).

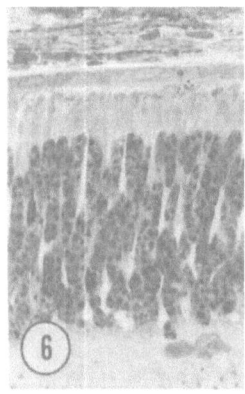 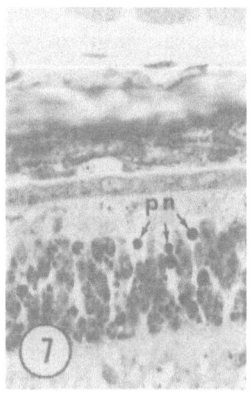 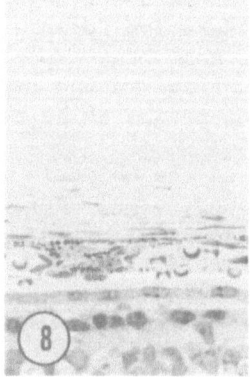

FIGURES 6-8. Retinas from rd/rd mutant mice showing progressive
    degeneration and disappearance of photoreceptor cells. Fig.
    6, 10 days of age; Fig. 7, day 13; Fig. 8, day 21. pn, pyk-
    notic nuclei. Epon-Araldite. One to 1.5 μm. Toluidine blue.
    X 600. Figures from LaVail and Sidman, *Arch. Ophthal.* 91:394-
    400 (1974). Reprinted with permission from the American Medi-
    cal Association, copyright 1974.

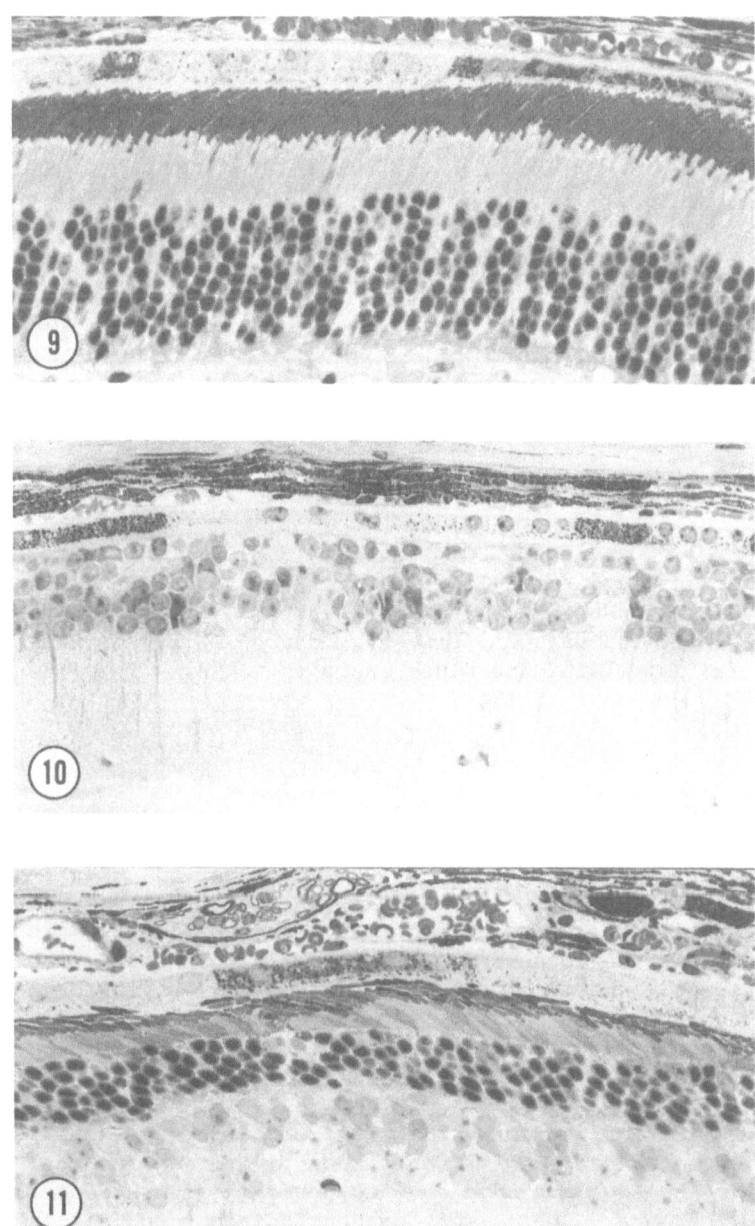

FIGURES 9-11. Retinas from three different mouse chimeras. Both
albino (<u>rd/rd</u>) and pigmented (+/+) pigment epithelial cells
are seen opposite normal (Fig. 9), degenerated (Fig. 10), and
intermediate (Fig. 11) retina. Epon-Araldite. One to 1.5 μm.
Toluidine blue. X 475.

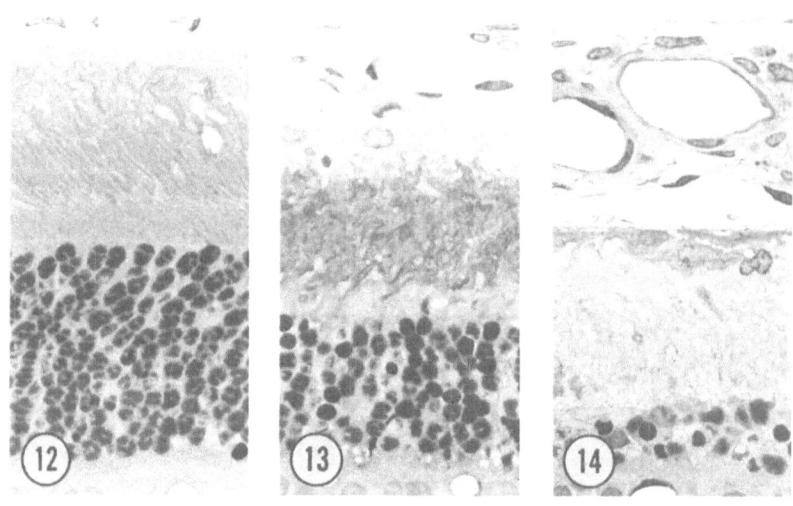

FIGURES 12-14. Retinas from rdy/rdy (RCS) mutant rats showing progressive disorganization of the rod outer segments and degeneration of photoreceptor cells. Figure 12, 20 days of age; Fig. 13, day 32; Fig. 14, day 44. Epon-Araldite. One to 1.5 μm. Toluidine blue. X 685.

We have produced two rat chimeras and have examined their eyes at different ages. The genotypes were rdy/rdy ↔ +/+ and rdy/rdy ↔ +/rdy (+/rdy heterozygotes have normal retinas). In both cases the rdy/rdy embryos were from the pink-eyed RCS strain, whose pigment epithelial cells appear non-pigmented by light microscopy of 1-2 μm plastic sections (Figs. 12-14). In both cases, the embryos with presumptive normal retinas were from fully pigmented strains. Therefore, the non-pigmented pigment epithelial cells carried the mutant genotype and the pigmented cells carried the normal genotype, as diagrammed in Fig. 5.

In the eye of a chimera taken at 26 days of age, outer segment debris was found adjacent to only non-pigmented rdy/rdy pigment epithelium and was not adjacent to normal, pigmented cells (Fig. 15). Furthermore, debris was present adjacent to all patches of rdy/rdy pigment epithelium greater than one or two cells in length.

The other three eyes of the two rat chimeras were taken at ages older than 100 days because the eyes were grossly pigmented, and we wished to examine the eyes when photoreceptor degeneration was complete. In each of the three eyes, patches of degenerating and degenerated photoreceptors were restricted to regions opposite

rdy/rdy pigment epithelial cells (Fig. 16-17). Some photoreceptor
cell loss was evident opposite all patches of mutant pigment epithelium greater than one or two cells in length.

    The finding of a direct correspondence of degenerating photo-
receptors with mutant pigment epithelium best fits the general
diagram in Fig. 5a and has led us to the conclusion that the site
of mutant gene expression in the rat disease is the pigment epithelial cell (Mullen and LaVail, 1976).   Additional observations
on the chimeric rat retinas will be described below with regard to
possible interactions among mutant and normal cells.

FURTHER CONSIDERATIONS OF THE CHIMERIC ANALYSIS

Identification of Photoreceptor Cell Genotypes

    Whereas pigmentation phenotype identifies the genotype of the
pigment epithelial cells in experimental chimeras, no direct marker
yet exists for identifying the genotype of photoreceptor cells. In
the case of the mouse chimeras, the genotype is implied by either
the survival (+/+) or disappearance (rd/rd) of the photoreceptor
cells. However, a question exists of the genotype of photoreceptor
cells in regions of intermediate retina. A direct cytochemical
marker to determine genotype would be useful because the interpretation of intermediate retina differs, depending upon the geno-
type(s) of the cells. If all the cells proved to be +/+ at the rd
locus, then the intermediate pattern must derive from intermingling
of +/+ and rd/rd cells during histogenesis or from displacement or
rearrangement   during degeneration of rd/rd cells or during subsequent growth of the eye. If, however, some of the photoreceptor
cells in intermediate retina proved to be surviving rd/rd cells,
then this would imply a retardation or block of the genetically
determined cell degeneration, presumably mediated by surrounding
cells. This would open the possibility of retarding or preventing
photoreceptor degeneration in the rd/rd mouse by identifying and
applying the mediating factor (see discussion in LaVail and Mullen,
1976).

    In the chimeric rats, we assume that an abnormality in the
mutant pigment epithelium causes the death of adjacent photoreceptor cells, regardless of their genotype. Here, we assume that both
genetically normal photoreceptor cells are present opposite genetically normal pigment epithelium, because the data from mouse
chimeras indicate that photoreceptors and pigment epithelium have
independent lineages (Mintz and Sanyal, 1970; Mintz, 1974). Nevertheless, a direct marker for the genotype of the photoreceptor
cells would be useful to confirm this assumption.

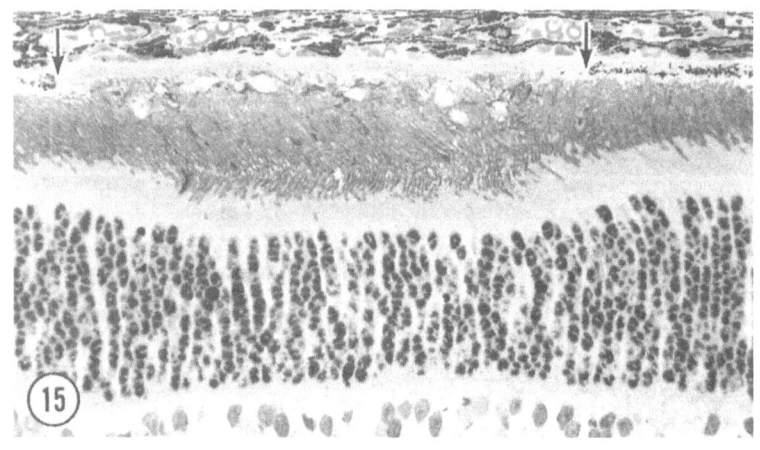

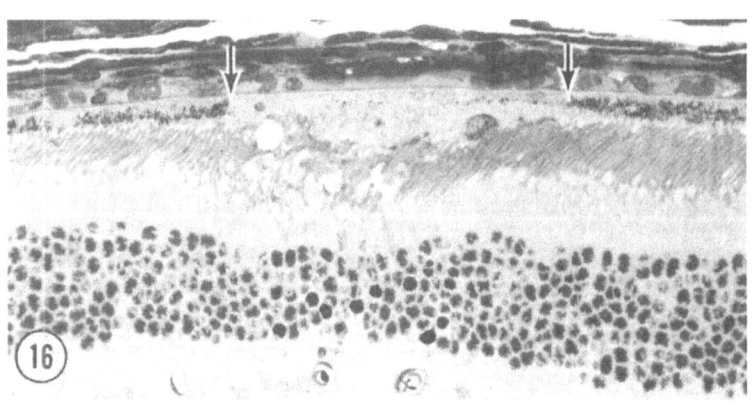

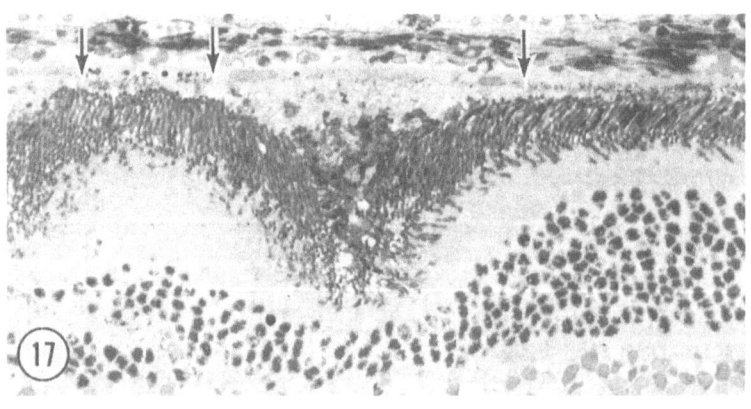

Cellular Localization of Mutant Gene Action

When no direct correlation of mutant pigment epithelium and degenerated retina is found in chimeras, as seen in the mouse chimeras (e.g., Fig. 5b), then two issues must be faced. First, the precise cellular localization of the mutant gene action cannot be directly determined at present. Although the pigment epithelium cell can be excluded (except see the second issue below), the cellular localization can only be to the neural retina and not to the photoreceptor per se. In all probability, the photoreceptor cell is the site of rd gene action, but some other cell might be involved (Blanks et al., 1974).

The second issue deals with gene pleiotropism, a rather common phenomenon in mammalian genetics. The possibility exists that the rd gene acts in a cell(s) remote from the eye, in addition to a cell within the neural retina. Based on the chimera data alone, the argument could be made that a circulating factor killed only rd/rd photoreceptor cells, thereby involving a pleitropic effect and giving a picture identical to Fig. 5b. However, the findings of Sidman (1961), who used organ culture studies, indicate that the genetic defect is intrinsic to the eye. The argument could further be made that the mutant pigment epithelium produces a widely diffusible substance that is toxic only to rd/rd photoreceptor cells (again, requiring a pleiotropic effect) which could result in a pattern such as that in Fig. 5b, instead of simply that in Fig. 5c. Evidence against this possibility comes from tissue culture experiments in which rd/rd neural retina was found to degenerate in the absence of the pigment epithelium (discussed in LaVail and Mullen, 1976). The point to be made is that if a positive correlation of mutant pigment epithelium and degenerating photoreceptors does not exist, as in the case of the mouse chimeras, the chimeric data

---

FIGURES 15-17. Retinas from rat chimeras illustrating accumulation of outer segment debris and loss of photoreceptor cell nuclei only adjacent to non-pigmented, rdy/rdy pigment epithelial cells and not adjacent to pigmented, normal pigment epithelial cells. In Figs. 15 and 16, the non-pigmented pigment epithelium is located between the two arrows; in Fig. 17, it is located to the left of the arrow on the left and between the center arrow and the arrow on the right. The number of melanosomes in pigment epithelial cells is smaller in the superior region of the eye, which explains the small number in the cells in Fig. 17. Numerous pyknotic nuclei are present in the patch of degenerating retina in Fig. 16. Figure 15, 26 days of age; Fig. 16, day 127; Fig. 17, day 111. Epon-Araldite. One to 1.5 μm. Toluidine blue. X 475.

alone cannot conclusively eliminate the possibility of pleiotropic effects.

Because of a positive correlation of mutant pigment epithelium and degenerating photoreceptors in the rat chimeras, we have concluded that the rdy gene in the rat acts in the pigment epithelial cell (Mullen and LaVail, 1976). This does not exclude the possibility that the rdy gene also acts in cells remote from the eye. For example, a circulating factor might be responsible for the pigment epithelial cell defect. However, this seems unlikely because such a factor would have to act only on rdy/rdy pigment epithelial cells, since only those pigment epithelial cells cause photoreceptor degeneration in the chimeras. Furthermore, the cells of origin of such a factor should themselves be present in diminished numbers (or be absent) because the tissues in which they reside presumably would also be chimeric. The supporting data to exclude this complex mechanism, such as organ and tissue culture experiments which remove the tissues from circulating factors (as described above for the mouse) do not exist, primarily because normal rat retina does not survive well in culture at ages much older than about 20 postnatal days (LaVail, unpublished observations). This last mechanism discussed here should be of less immediate concern unless future experiments with isolated pigment epithelium fail to show differences between mutant and normal control tissues, and even then the presence or absence of interacting photoreceptors must still be considered.

Possible Interactions Among Mutant and Normal Cells

One biologically interesting feature unique to the study of experimental chimeras is that cells of different genotypes are brought together in a physiological environment. New cell interactions are made possible that can be obtained in no other way. The insights provided by these interactions may suggest the mechanism and potential treatment of retinal degenerations. One example, discussed above, is the possibility that interaction of rd/rd and +/+ photoreceptor cells in chimeric mice produce intermediate retina, perhaps by prolonging the survival of rd/rd cells.

In chimeric rat retinas, the following observations suggest that interactions do occur between mutant and normal cells: (1) in all but one patch of mutant pigment epithelium, the extent of photoreceptor degeneration was less than expected for the age of the animal (Fig. 16); (2) there was usually little cell death opposite small patches of one or two mutant pigment epithelial cells; and (3) rod outer segments usually were less disorganized at the periphery of patches of mutant pigment epithelium (Mullen and LaVail, 1976). The simplest interpretation of these findings is that the adjacent, normal pigment epithelial cells supply some nutrient or metabolite to the photoreceptors that the mutant pigment epithelial cells lack. Furthermore, in a preliminary electron microscopic study, two unexpected phagosomes were recognized in a rdy/rdy pigment epithelial cell that was close to +/+ pigment epithelial cells near the periphery of a patch. Further work is needed to determine whether phagocytosis by mutant pigment epithelial cells, which usually do not phagocytize outer segment discs, is a common finding in these chimeras. If so, it suggests that normal pigment epithelial cells may provide a substance, perhaps a surface recognition factor for outer segment discs, which would allow for phagocytosis that is ordinarily missing in rdy/rdy pigment epithelial cells. The findings discussed here give some hope that retinal dystrophy in the rat can be retarded or prevented if the mediating factor(s) can be identified and isolated.

Indices of Retinal Mosaicism

As a practical matter, it would be desirable to be able to predict whether a given retina displays much (or any) mosaicism if, for example, expensive radioisotopes are to be injected or lengthy behavioral studies are to be carried out. We considered two features that might easily be used if they were good indices of retinal mosaicism--coat color and the pattern of retinal mosaicism of one eye (using the other for experimental purposes). To test these, we examined the coat colors of the chimeric mice used in the study by LaVail and Mullen (1976) and compared them to the degree of mosaicism in the pigment epithelium and in the neural retina of the two eyes of each of the animals. The approximate proportions of the different pigment epithelial and retinal phenotypes in one meridional section from each eye were recorded, and the pigment epithelium was scored as being either predominantly one phenotype (albino or pigmented), predominantly one phenotype but with numerous cells of the other phenotype, or a good mixture of the two phenotypes. The neural retina was scored similarly but for three phenotypes--normal, degenerated, and intermediate. Retina and pigment epithelium were said to be similar, for example, if the pigment epithelium of an SJL ↔ B10 chimera was mostly albino (rd/rd) with only a few pigmented cells, and the retina was mostly degenerated (presumed rd/rd) with only a few patches classed as intermediate or normal. For this comparison only, intermediate retina and rd/rd pigmented epithelium were said to be similar, because intermediate retina may be the result of rd/rd photoreceptors having originally been present amongst +/+ cells. The percent of albino coat color was determined at weaning (Mullen and Whitten, 1971).

The results are presented in Table I. While the data can give only a crude estimate because only one section through each eye was scored, they indicate that a strikingly high percentage of the mice

TABLE I

COMPARISON OF THE DEGREE OF MOSAICISM IN PIGMENT EPITHELIUM, NEURAL RETINA, AND COAT COLOR IN CHIMERIC MICE*

	Strain Combinations***		
	SJL↔B10	C3H↔BALB	SJL↔B10CBAF₁
Pigment epithelium and neural retina similar in individual eyes	38/41 eyes	17/19 eyes	11/13 eyes
Pigment epithelium and neural retina similar in the two eyes of individual mice**	16/17 mice	6/6 mice	6/6 mice
If coat color is 1–20% or 80–99% albino, retina and pigment epithelium mostly like the predominant coat color (others more patchy)**	6/8 mice	8/9 mice	5/5 mice
If coat color is 25–75% albino, retina and pigment epithelium patchy (others predominantly one phenotype)**	4/9 mice	0/3 mice	2/2 mice

*Criteria for comparison given in text. Mice from the study of LaVail and Mullen (1976).

**Animals were not counted in which the pigment epithelium was dissimilar to the retina in one of the eyes.

***These are abbreviations for the following inbred strains with their respective genotypes at the rd and albino, c, loci: SJL/J (rd/rd c/c); C57BL/10GnDg (+/+ +/+); C3H/HeJ (rd/rd, +/+); BALB/cGnDgWt (+/+ c/c). The B10CBAF₁ abbreviation indicates that these embryos were F₁ hybrids of the C57BL/10GnDg and CBA/J (rd/rd +/+) strains and therefore had the genotype +/rd +/+.

had similar degrees of mosaicism in the two eyes. Therefore, the
histology of one eye would probably yield a fairly accurate picture
of the histology of the second eye.

Coat color provides a somewhat less good index of retinal
mosaicism (Table I). If the coat color is 80% or greater of one
phenotype, the chances are good that the retina and pigment epithelium are predominantly of the same corresponding phenotypes.
However, if the coat color is very patchy, with 25-75% of one
phenotype, the degree of retinal mosaicism appears to be unpredic-
table. On the other hand, most examples of very patchy retinas
will be found in those chimeras with a very patchy coat color.

FUTURE APPLICATION OF EXPERIMENTAL CHIMERAS IN VISION RESEARCH

Experimental chimeras are a powerful tool with which to
analyze the role of the pigment epithelium in inherited retinal
degenerations. If technically feasible, the chimeric analysis
should be applied to all retinal degenerations in laboratory
animals. There need not be an obvious suggestion of pigment epithelial cell involvement, such as the presence of outer segment
debris in the RCS rat, to warrant questioning the role of the
pigment epithelium in retinal degenerations. The pigment epithelium plays many other roles in addition to that involved in outer
segment renewal in maintaining the normal physiology of photoreceptor cells, including metabolic transport (see review in Young and
Bok, 1976), ion transport (Lasansky and de Fisch, 1965; Steinberg
and Miller, 1973), synthesis of some of the interphotoreceptor
matrix (Berman, 1964; Feeney, 1973) and vitamin A metabolism
(Dowling, 1960; Zimmerman, 1974). It is possible that dysfunction
of any of these metabolic processes could produce photoreceptor
degeneration without the appearance or accumulation of outer segment debris.

The question of future use of chimeras in vision research,
therefore, revolves around two factors that affect technical feasibility. First, appropriate pigmentation phenotypes or other types
of cell markers must be available to distinguish pigment epithelial
cell genotypes, and second, one must be able to make chimeras with
embryos of a given species. Clearly, any mouse mutation can be
analyzed with chimeras, and we soon will be using chimeras to study
the new forms of retinal degeneration in Purkinje cell degeneration, pcd, and nervous, nr, mice described by Mullen and LaVail
(1975). Rat chimeras have proved more difficult to produce than
mouse chimeras (Mullen and LaVail, 1976). However, when a positive
correlation exists between mutant pigment epithelium and degenerating retina, as in the case with the rat chimeras, considerable
information can be obtained from just a few animals. Although production of chimeras of even larger animals may be more difficult,

chimeric rabbits (Gardner and Munro, 1974; Moustafa, 1974) and chimeric sheep (Tucker *et al.*, 1974) have recently been produced by a slightly different technique than that used by us for rodent chimeras. Thus, the technology exists for producing chimeras of perhaps all mammalian species. Furthermore, the successful freezing, storage and subsequent transplantation of embryos has been accomplished (Whittingham and Whitten, 1974). If this technology can be used with embryos of larger species, it would obviate the need for simultaneous matings and might facilitate the application of the chimeric analysis of retinal degenerations to those laboratory animals.

ACKNOWLEDGMENTS

This work was supported in part by USPHS Research Grant EY-01202 (M.M.L.) and Research Career Development Award EY-70871 (M.M.L.) from the National Eye Institute and by a Basil O'Connor Starter Research Grant from the National Foundation-March of Dimes (R.J.M.).

REFERENCES

Aguirre, G., and Rubin, L. F. (1976) Animal model systems with disorders of the retinal pigment epithelium, in "The Retinal Pigment Epithelium" (K. M. Zinn and M. F. Marmor, eds.) Harvard University Press, Cambridge (In press).

Berman, E. R. (1964) The biosynthesis of mucopolysaccharides and glycoproteins in pigment epithelial cells of bovine retina. *Biochim. Biophys. Acta* 83:371-373.

Blanks, J. C., Adinolfi, A. M., and Lolley, R. N. (1974) Photoreceptor degeneration and synaptogenesis in retinal-degenerative (rd) mice. *J. Comp. Neurol.* 156:95-106.

Bok, D., and Hall, M. O. (1971) The role of the pigment epithelium in the etiology of inherited retinal dystrophy in the rat. *J. Cell Biol.* 49:664-682.

Burden, E. M., Yates, C. M., Reading, H. W., Bitensky, L., and Chayen, J. (1971) Investigation into the structural integrity of lysosomes in the normal and dystrophic rat retina. *Exp. Eye Res.* 12:159-165.

Dowling, J. E. (1960) Chemistry of visual adaptation in the rat. *Nature (London)* 188:114-118.

Farber, D. B., and Lolley, R. N. (1974) Cyclic guanosine monophosphate: elevation in degenerating photoreceptor cells of the C3H mouse retina. *Science* 186:449-451.

Feeney, L. (1973) Synthesis of interphotoreceptor matrix. I. Autoradiography of ^{3}H-fucose incorporation. *Invest. Ophthal.* 12: 739-751.

Gardner, R. L., and Munro, A. J. (1974) Successful construction of chimaeric rabbit. *Nature* 250:146-147.

Herron, W. L., Jr., Riegel, B. W., Myers, O. E., and Rubin, M. L. (1969) Retinal dystrophy in the rat--a pigment epithelial disease. *Invest. Ophthal.* 8:595-604.

Lasansky, A., and de Fisch, F. W. (1965) Studies on the function of the pigment epithelium in relation to ionic movement between retina and choroid, in "The Structure of the Eye. II. Symposium" (J. W. Rohen, ed.) Schattauer-Verlag, Stuttgart.

LaVail, M. M. (1976) The pigment epithelium in mice and rats with inherited retinal degeneration, in "The Retinal Pigment Epithelium" (K. M. Zinn and M. F. Marmor, eds). Harvard University Press, Cambridge (In press).

LaVail, M. M., and Mullen, R. J. (1976) Role of the pigment epithelium in inherited retinal degeneration analyzed with experimental mouse chimeras. *Exp. Eye Res.* 23:227-245.

LaVail, M. M., and Sidman, R. L. (1974) C57BL/6J mice with inherited retinal degeneration. *Arch. Ophthal.* 91:394-400.

Lolley, R. N. (1973) RNA and DNA in developing retinae: comparison of a normal with the degenerating retinae of C3H mice. *J. Neurochem.* 20:175-182.

Mintz, B. (1962) Formation of genotypically mosaic mouse embryos. *Amer. Zool.* 2:432.

Mintz, B. (1964) Formation of genetically mosaic mouse embryos, and early development of "lethal (t^{12}/t^{12})-normal" mosaics. *J. Exp. Zool.* 157:273-292.

Mintz, B. (1965) Genetic mosaicism in adult mice of quadriparental lineage. *Science* 148:1232-1233.

Mintz, B. (1974) Gene control of mammalian differentiation. *Ann. Rev. Genet.* 8:411-470.

Mintz, B., and Sanyal, S. (1970) Clonal origin of the mouse visual retina mapped from genetically mosaic eyes. *Genetics* (Suppl.) 64:43-44.

Moustafa, L. A. (1974) Chimaeric rabbits from embryonic cell transplantation. *Proc. Soc. Exp. Biol. Med.* 147:485-488.

Mullen, R. J., and LaVail, M. M. (1975) Two new types of retinal degeneration in cerebellar mutant mice. *Nature (London)* 258: 528-530.

Mullen, R. J., and LaVail, M. M. (1976) Inherited retinal dystrophy: primary defect in pigment epithelium determined with experimental rat chimeras. *Science* 192:799-801.

Mullen, R. J., and Whitten, W. K. (1971) Relationship of genotype and degree of chimerism in coat color to sex ratios and gametogenesis in chimeric mice. *J. Exp. Zool.* 178:165-176.

Sanyal, S., and Bal, A. K. (1973) Comparative light and electron microscopic study of retinal histogenesis in normal and rd mutant mice. *Z. Anat. Entwickl.-Gesch.* 142:219-238.

Schmidt, S. Y., and Lolley, R. N. (1973) Cyclic-nucleotide phosphodiesterase. An early defect in inherited retinal degeneration of C3H mice. *J. Cell Biol.* 57:117-123.

Sidman, R. L. (1961) Tissue culture studies of inherited retinal dystrophy. *Dis. Nerv. System* 22:14-20.

Steinberg, R. H., and Miller, S. (1973) Aspects of electrolyte transport in frog pigment epithelium. *Exp. Eye Res.* 16:365-372.

Tarkowski, A. K. (1961) Mouse chimaeras developed from fused eggs. *Nature (London)* 190:857-860.

Tucker, E. M., Moor, R. M., and Rowson, L. E. A. (1974) Tetraparental sheep chimaeras induced by blastomere transplantation. *Immunol.* 26:613-621.

Wegmann, T. G., LaVail, M. M., and Sidman, R. L. (1971) Patchy retinal degeneration in tetraparental mice. *Nature (London)* 230:333-334.

Whittingham, D. G., and Whitten, W. K. (1974) Long-term storage and aerial transport of frozen mouse embryos. *J. Reprod. Fert.* 36:433-435.

Young, R. W., and Bok, D. (1976) Metabolism of the pigment epithe-
     lium, in "The Retinal Pigment Epithelium" (K. M. Zinn and
     M. F. Marmor, eds.) Harvard University Press, Cambridge (In
     press).

Zimmerman, W. F. (1974)   The distribution and proportions of vita-
     min A compounds during the visual cycle in the rat. *Vis. Res.*
     14:795-802.

DISCUSSION OF THE PAPER

DR. HERRON: I just want to congratulate Dr. LaVail on an
absolutely beautiful paper.

DR. LAVAIL: Thank you, Warren.

DR. LATIES: In my brief introduction I mentioned to you how
important it is to find out the locus of activity and I think that
is the essence of Dr. LaVail's paper. He has moved us a great distance in these studies in finding out where we have to look further
to find out what is happening.

CORTICAL REPRESENTATION OF RETINAL DEGENERATION

Werner K. Noell

Neurosensory Laboratory
University of Buffalo
Buffalo, New York

(Summary by M. L. Wolbarsht from conference recording)

Previous work has been done by Matthew LaVail and his associates on the visual capacities of rats after the degeneration of the visual cells as documented by both conventional histology and electron microscopy of the retina. Two of my associates, Mr. Marty Silensky and Mr. Richard Stockton and I have extended the work with some electrophysiological measurements on the cortex and the optic tract. The skull was opened to record from the left hemisphere of the brain. Electrodes were put at different places in the visual cortex while stimulating with diffuse light. This stimulates all the various points on the surface of the cerebral cortex which represent the visual field--the horizontal meridian, vertical, straightforward, nasal, temporal, 40° in the lower field and 40° in the upper visual field, as later documented by small spot stimulation. Long-haired pigmented hereditary dystrophic rats were used with normal rats as controls. Computer averaging of the visual evoked potentials was used, although individual potentials were recorded as large as 1.2 millivolts. These are similar to the same type of recording in humans with a positive downward deflection P_1 and N_1, and an upward negative deflection followed with a slow wave. In the normal response, P_1 is the activity of the incoming systems. This early input to the visual cortex occurs in about 40-50 milliseconds after the flash and is the excitatory component. There is a relatively brief post-synaptic potential in the cerebral cortex which is completed within 50 milliseconds after the flash. This indicated a fairly synchronous type of activity. The response disappears if the light intensity is reduced one or two log units. This is strong light response and is accompanied by normal ERG's.

In hereditary dystrophic rats, 55 days after birth the ERG's are about 50 microvolts as compared with 250 microvolts in the normal rats, a reduction of about five times. At 125 days the ERG, even with computer averaging, is almost absent in the dystrophic rats. This indicates a degeneration of the retina associated with loss of visual cells and debris accumulation. The evoked potential at the age of 53 days is almost normal. The latency is slightly increased, and the response comes mainly from the periphery of the visual field where the visual cells tend to survive the longest. They certainly definitely are still alive at this time. At 277 days after birth the visual cortex still has a response. The response is to flashes of light--not noise or smell. The retina without visual cells has an excitatory response which activates the visual cortex. Stimulation in the center of the visual field in albino rats where there are no outer segments preserved also gives a maximum response. At 260 days the ERG of the dystrophic rat is virtually absent with a b-wave which comes a bit later than the first response in the cortex. This shows that there is a visual cortex response stimulation of a blind retina confirming the psychophysical data of LaVail and others who were not believed, including those workers in the 1920's who used mice. A litter which at 288 days is half normal and half abnormal makes it easy to compare the electroretinograms and cortical responses of the abnormal with the normal. The cortical response from the normals averaged 100 millivolts for a single flash. The abnormal litter mate had essentially the same response, a little bit reduced in the periphery, but not in the center. The responses remain at reduced intensities. The threshold is elevated less than three log units even after 120 to 150 days, at which time the ERG is flat. Something gets out of the retina with a greatly increased latency.

The important question is what generates this excitatory response in the degenerated retina. How is light transduced into excitation? Is it from the few visual cells which survive in the periphery near the ora serrata or is it in some remnants of the photoreceptor cells? Often one row of cone nuclei remains, sometimes with a few relatively short inner segments. Our recordings from the optic tracts furnish some information. Normally a single unit in the optic tract which responds when the center of its receptive field is illuminated (center on) has an inhibitory off response. The surround is the opposite and the response latency is about 25 milliseconds. Even in a 196 day old rat, on-center cells can be found and they are relatively more common than in a normal. The latency is slightly longer but these cells still have a very fast and vigorous response with over 500 impulses per second. The retinas were examined in serial section from the animals with good cortical recordings. There were visual cells only in the very peripheral region next to the ora serrata, so far out that it was not even represented in our cortical map. In these retinas all of the outer segments, and the outer nuclear layer except for one row of nuclei, had disappeared. In a small area there were inner segments with no outer segments. In this region, light stimulation gave excitation with a cortical response.

In the retina of an animal 85 days old there is much debris and only one row of nuclei still survive. These are probably cones, as they are very resistant to degeneration. Even they tend to disappear in older animals.   Their nuclei are pycnotic, and it is probably these cells whose visual capacity LaVail was measuring. These cells don't seem to have any visual pigment to transduce light into nervous energy.   Still, there is a normal response in the cerebral cortex. Light exposure which destroys only two-thirds of the retina gives no response to stimulation in regions of no visual cells; where there are good visual cells there is a good response.   However, in the complete destruction of the retina, inner segments only are sufficient for a response.   The outer seg-ments don't seem to be needed. LaVail has made the point that synaptic network is intact in these retinas and that there is no abnormality except that the cone cells have fewer synaptic endings with bipolar cells than in normal retinas.

There is another problem--that the information which comes out of the retina must be magnified within the cortex in an abnor-mal way.   This must be some sort of plasticity reaction of the cerebral cortex.   The cerebral cortex determines and compensates for the natural changes.   The cerebral cortex then responds plas-tically with time to this lowered input from the retina. The rat lives with a visual abnormality in dim or very dim light and tries to make the best sense out of what he has left in his visual system.

DISCUSSION OF THE PAPER

DR. WOLBARSHT: I don't think there is any plasticity and I am not surprised at your results. I will explain what I mean by that. When you do electrophysiology of the retina of any animal, and the rat is no exception, you find that the connections to any ganglion cell from the retina includes a very large area of the retina. Indeed, what you have labeled the surround is, as far as anybody has ever been able to document, the whole retina.   The anatomical connections support the physiological indications that there are enormous areas of convergence on ganglion cells from all directions in the retina.   Now, that is only the retina.   Further up in the visual system, there are even larger areas of summation. Generally they are not seen because of the interplay between excitation and inhibition that results in only a small receptive field actually seen at the cortex when everything is working.   The minute that cells begin to drop out things from this interplay, the more peri-pheral regions are seen.   These usually get choked off by the stronger representations from the central areas. I would not be surprised that if only one receptor was left most of the cortex would be activated. There is nothing plastic about that; the connections were always there.

DR. NOELL: The evidence is against that as I showed in the last slide. I make much less damage in the normal adult than in the hereditary animal where it starts very early. There is nothing in those cortical regions which were connected to the retina without visual cells.

DR. WOLBARSHT: Well, now, wait a minute. There is a difference in their development which is pointed out by the experiments of Hubel and Wiesel, and Guillary. The developing nervous system will lose connections if there are not strong inputs to them. The connections start out the same originally and, let's say, are cemented together by use. Now, ablation of the retina in an adult would give a different pattern than in a developing animal. What you should look at is acute light exposure damage in an adult animal versus a chronic lesion in an adult animal. I think that you will see that there is very little difference.

DR. NOELL: There is even a difference in the mouse. The mouse undergoes this whole degeneration much faster than the rat, much faster. The mouse doesn't have time for the plasticity.

DR. STEPHENS: How much is the time differential between the retinal and the brain response in the rat during normal development?

DR. NOELL: The fast component in the brain response occurs about 15-20 milliseconds after the retinal response.

CURRENT TRENDS IN THERAPY: THEORY AND PRACTICE

INTRODUCTION

Myron L. Wolbarsht and Maurice B. Landers

Duke University Eye Center
Durham, North Carolina   27710

As our knowledge has increased from current research, we have reached a point where clinical applications may be considered. Although many animal models have been proposed, identification of any form of retinitis pigmentosa with any particular animal model is highly conjectural. For the researcher to suggest that his laboratory manipulations of an animal model can be applied immediately to the clinical management of retinitis pigmentosa is premature. For the clinician to accept such a suggestion, even on the most carefully selected patients, is to build up hopes that cannot possibly be fulfilled at the present.

At least one animal model of retinitis pigmentosa is related to the broader problem of the reaction of the human organism to the physical stresses of the normal environment. It is obvious that exposure to light levels in which natural safeguards, such as blinking, pain, tearing, etc., are overcome, will result in damage to the eye. Permanent damage of the retina can result from chronic exposures to high light intensity; at even higher intensities, there is actual degeneration of the retina. It has been long suspected that some cataracts result from chronic exposures to the ultraviolet and near infrared portions of sunlight. Similar changes occur in other parts of the body, such as the skin cancers in blondes exposed to too much ultraviolet sunlight. It is possible that other diseases, including retinitis pigmentosa, may result from the exaggerated sensitivity of certain individuals to the normal environmental stresses. The hypothesis that retinitis pigmentosa is an increase (of a hereditary nature) in sensitivity to

environmental light has made the basis for several types of therapy
ranging from complete occlusion of one eye to optical filters.
However, all of these still await careful evaluation on the basis
of large clinical trials.

When this symposium was organized, we felt it would not be out
of place to indicate how retinitis pigmentosa fitted into the more
general problem of hereditary eye diseases and the particular problems that they present to state health agencies. The indications
that therapy may be available for some particular untreatable and
uncontrolled eye diseases, of which again, retinitis pigmentosa is
one example, could further modify the public health problem.

RETINITIS PIGMENTOSA: CLINICAL MANAGEMENT BASED ON CURRENT

CONCEPTS

M. L. Wolbarsht, M. B. Landers, III, J. A. C. Wadsworth,
and W. B. Anderson, Jr.

Duke University Eye Center
Durham, North Carolina 27710

INTRODUCTION

Retinitis pigmentosa (RP) is the term used to describe a group of hereditary degenerative diseases of the retina. It is common-- the overall incidence may be as high as 0.5%. In this condition pigment clumps resembling bone spicules accumulate within the retina. This is followed by an attenuation of the retinal vessels and optic atrophy. The disease is progressive, often manifesting itself first in childhood and leading to complete blindness before the age of 50. Night blindness and progressive limitation of the visual field are often preceded by an almost complete disappearance of the electroretinogram (ERG). Occasionally the disappearance of the ERG is stepwise with the rod portion diminishing first. The earliest symptoms of retinitis pigmentosa are an impairment in dark adaptation and a loss of peripheral vision. As these are also the earliest ocular symptoms encountered in chronic vitamin A deficiency, it has been suggested that a specific therapy for retinitis pigmentosa might be high doses of vitamin A (Dowling and Gibbons, 1961). However, there are indications that this therapy is of no apparent value (Chatzinoff *et al.*, 1968; Bergsma and Wolf, 1977). We indicate a rationale for this failure and even suggest that vitamin A intake should be minimized or eliminated for a short time.

This hypothesis is based on information from an animal model, the so-called "dystrophic" rat, which resembles in many ways the human disease. In the dystrophic rat the easy availability of vitamin A appears to accelerate the course of the disease (Dowling and Wald, 1960), while severe restriction of vitamin A intake may inhibit some phases of the disease (Herron and Riegel, 1974). In the animal model the normal course of the disease is accelerated by light and elevated retinal (or body) temperature (Noell *et al.*, 1966).

SIMILARITY BETWEEN RP AND RETINAL DYSTROPHY IN RATS

Although definite proof is lacking, retinitis pigmentosa is at present considered to be similar to the form of hereditary retinal dystrophy in the RCS strain of dystrophic rats (Feeney, 1973). In these rats, exposure to light produces retinal dystrophy in which the retina may almost completely degenerate in a few days. The dystrophy occurs even if the rats are kept in nearly total darkness, but with a much slower time course. The disappearance of the ERG is the earliest sign. In the animal model one feature of the disease is an accumulation of rod outer segments. In a normal rat retina the rod outer segments continue to grow during life and are continually phagocytized by pigment epithelium in order to keep the length of the outer segment constant. The outer segments of the cones apparently do not grow after their initial differentiation (Young, 1973). This balance between rod outer segment length and phagocytosis is disturbed in rats with inherited retinal dystrophy in such a way that the rod outer segment growth relative to the rate of phagocytosis is increased and a large amount of rod outer segment material accumulates as retinal debris (Noell *et al.*, 1966; Feeney, 1973). Following this accumulation the retina degenerates, although the cause of the retinal degeneration is unknown. In humans with RP, the rods are severely affected first, accompanied by less severe manifestations in the cones (Berson and Howard, 1971). Some cone function may be retained after the rods have degenerated. This survival of cone function is probably responsible for the persistence of vision following retinal degeneration in humans as well as in rats (O'Steen and Anderson, 1971; Bennett *et al.*, 1973). In late stages of RP even the surviving cones (those in the fovea) may show some signs of abnormality, albeit they are still functional (Kolb and Gouras, 1974).

It is possible that in human RP patients, as well as in dystrophic rats, the accumulated rod outer segment debris, mostly lipid in nature, forms a diffusion barrier between the neural retina and both the pigment epithelium and the choroidal circulation. This would be, in effect, a retinal detachment and could lead to a degeneration of the outer retina in a similar fashion.

Anderson (1968) has shown that the time to blackout in normal human subjects following an increase in intraocular pressure to levels above arterial supply pressure is a simple function of blood oxygenation. Prebreathing 100% oxygen, as compared with normal air (20% oxygen), markedly increases the time to blackout and the time

to complete recovery of function following the blackout is correspondingly decreased. Retinitis pigmentosa patients, however, do
not show as markedly the increased time to blackout. We interpret
these results as indicating the presence in the RP patient of an
increased metabolic demand or a smaller oxygen reservoir, either
or both of which could be coupled with a diffusion barrier, such
as the rod outer segment debris between the choroidal circulation
and the photoreceptor layer of the retina.   In addition, it is
possible that the accumulated detached rod outer segment discs are
still functional. This could place an additional metabolic demand
upon the dissolved oxygen in the diffusion pathway, thus further
lowering the oxygen available to the photoreceptors.

The degeneration of the retina may be accelerated by an aller-
gic response. For example, Char *et al*. (1974) have shown that .the
patients with retinal pigment degeneration (of various types,
including retinitis pigmentosa) showed a cell mediated immunity to
retinoblastoma cells which was much higher than that in normal subjects. This suggests that cellular immune processes may play a
role in the pathogenesis or pathophysiology of retinitis pigmentosa, as well as other types of retinal degeneration. After they
are initiated by other factors, these immune reactions may amplify
(or add to) these degenerations.

Other pathological changes may also be possible in response
to one or more of the many stages of the retinal degeneration process, set in progress by the original imbalance between the rate of
rod outer segment growth and the rate of phagocytosis. However,
the initial cause of retinal dystrophy in rats appears to be an
imbalance between rod outer segment accumulation and the rate of
phagocytosis by the pigment epithelium. The greater the imbalance
the more rapidly the disease progresses; the smaller the imbalance
the more slowly the disease progresses. Thus, factors which
accelerate rod outer segment growth should be minimized in order
to slow or arrest the progress of the disease. On the other hand,
factors which would tend to retard normal growth of the rod outer
segment should be emphasized. It is even possible that complete
destruction of the rods, that is, converting the retina to an all-
cone system, may arrest the disease, leaving the cone function more
or less intact. Factors which accelerate rod outer segment production should increase the disparity between rod outer segment growth
and the subsequent phagocytosis by the pigment epithelium and could
produce pathologic processes in normal retina if carried to excess.
Many factors have been suggested to account for the imbalance,
although any single one may be sufficient to explain it.

It is most likely that in retinitis pigmentosa, several factors may operate more or less independently of each other and the
specific different genetic makeups may each control a single factor. However, each of the factors operates to create an imbalance

between rod outer segment growth and its subsequent phagocytosis by the pigment epithelium. The possible factors are: hyperplasia, or overactivity of the rod with regard to the outer segment growth; improper maturation of the rod outer segment with regard to the development of a recognition factor to activate the phagosomes in the pigment epithelium at the proper time; and some defect in the phagosomes, such as hypoactivity. Tests on the pigment epithelium of RCS rats indicate normal phagosome activity with regard to many types of substances other than rod outer segment material (Feeney, 1973). Thus, the recognition factor (Herron *et al.*, 1974) or hyperactivity of rod outer segment growth appear to be the more likely causes. Of course, in the areas of the retina where the rods are the predominant photoreceptors, the debris accumulates the most rapidly. For this reason, the peripheral portions of the retina where the rods far outnumber the cones are affected first. In the fovea and parafoveal regions, where the rods are few or nonexistent, sight is retained longest. It is even possible that the gradual progressive loss of macular function, including even the rod-free fovea, may be due to a secondary atrophy of the inner layers of the retina following the disappearance of retinal blood vessels.

RATIONALE FOR THERAPY

In the rat the course of the disease is also accelerated by exposure to light (Noell *et al.*, 1966), by elevated body temperature (Noell *et al.*, 1966), and also by the easy availability of vitamin A (Dowling and Gibbons, 1961), and the essential fatty acids utilized in rod outer segment growth (Landis *et al.*, 1973). On the other hand, restriction of vitamin A inhibits rod outer segment formation while apparently sparing the cones (Dowling and Wald, 1960; Herron and Riegel, 1974).

Exposure to Visible Light

Light is the major stimulus to rod outer segment formation. In the dystrophic rats normal amounts of light cause early retinal degeneration; darkness inhibits the onset (Noell *et al.*, 1966; Gorn and Kuwabara, 1967; Young, 1973). Even in normal animals, long term exposure to higher than normal photic stresses will result in retinal pathology (Lawwill, 1973; Tso, 1973). This may indicate that retinitis pigmentosa is an exaggerated sensitivity to activation of rod outer segment formation by light, or possibly even deactivation by light of the phagosomal system of the pigment epithelium.

Berson (1971) has suggested the use of an occluder to prevent light from reaching the retina in one eye in patients with retinitis pigmentosa. The occluded eye will then be kept in reserve for use when the vision in the other eye has deteriorated below the useful level. However, it may be only necessary to prevent light from stimulating the rods. If this could be done while still permitting enough light to enter the eye for useful vision by the cones, then both eyes might be protected simultaneously. This could be done by using a filter whose absorption spectrum is closely matched to the action spectrum of rhodopsin. Since the main sensitivity of the cone system is at a longer wavelength than that of the rhodopsin (580 nm vs. 500 nm), a filter matched to the rod system should allow sufficient light to enter the eye to activate the cones without markedly stimulating the rods to produce outer segments. Rats exposed to red light for short periods each day, or rats left in total darkness do not develop retinal degeneration (Noell, private communication). Retinitis pigmentosa has a much slower time course for the disease as compared with that in the dystrophic rat--years as against days. The elimination of any rod production stimulus might greatly decrease or even arrest the progress of the disease. Formation of a rod outer segment with a slow enough rate may not result in a serious problem with regard to the amount of retinal debris.

The selection of a filter to exclude the proper portion of the spectrum is difficult. Figure 1 shows the absorption spectrum of rhodopsin as compared with other filters. The match between the spectacle lenses Glendale RP-1 and RP-B filters and rhodopsin is fairly good; the others are not quite as good. We are investigating the possibility of obtaining a more suitable type of plastic. These filters cut out much of the blue light, even more of the green, but very little of the yellow and red light. Thus, the light coming through the filter will appear subjectively to be yellow, as in Glendale RP-1 (or bronze, as in Glendale RP-B, if the near infrared is excluded as suggested below).

A proper test for the effectiveness of any filter is the dark adaptation that it induces in the rod system in use. The ideal filter should have a high visual efficiency under photic conditions, while blocking all light to the rod system. The amount of dark adaptation for several filters is shown in Fig. 2. The filter selected would also be useful as a dark adaptation filter for normal eyes.

Berson et al. (1973) have also proposed the use of a low level, night vision aid (similar to a sniper scope) for patients whose retina has been severely affected to increase the light intensity to levels where useful vision is attained. Following this line of reasoning, we suggest that any light amplifier device or sniper scope (Berson et al., 1973) should have a display screen

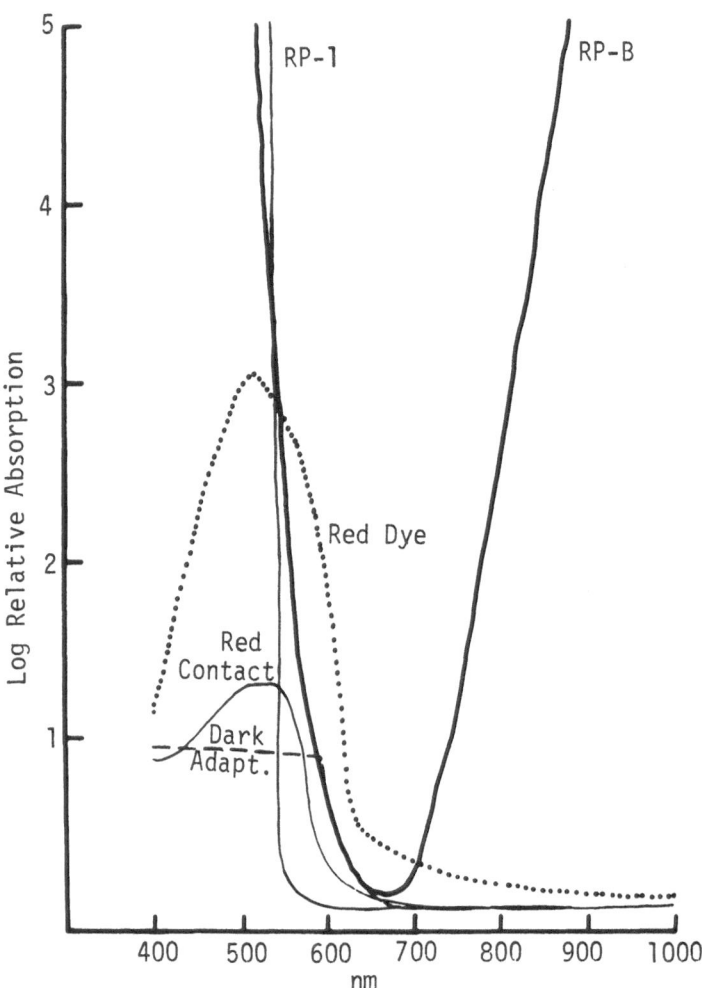

FIGURE 1. Comparative absorption spectra of filters used in retinitis pigmentosa therapy. The absorption is plotted relative
to air at unity absorption. RP-1 and RP-B are amber and
bronze spectacles, respectively, from Glendale Optical Company. The visual efficiency of these filters is between 40-
50%. The red dye filter is the standard plastic used in prescription spectacles treated with Basic Red Dye by White
Optical Company. The red contact filter is a Special Red
contact lens from Milton Roy Company. The dark adapt filter
is a commercial dark adaptation filter (American Cyanamid Red
R8613-80) with a visual efficiency of approximately 15%.

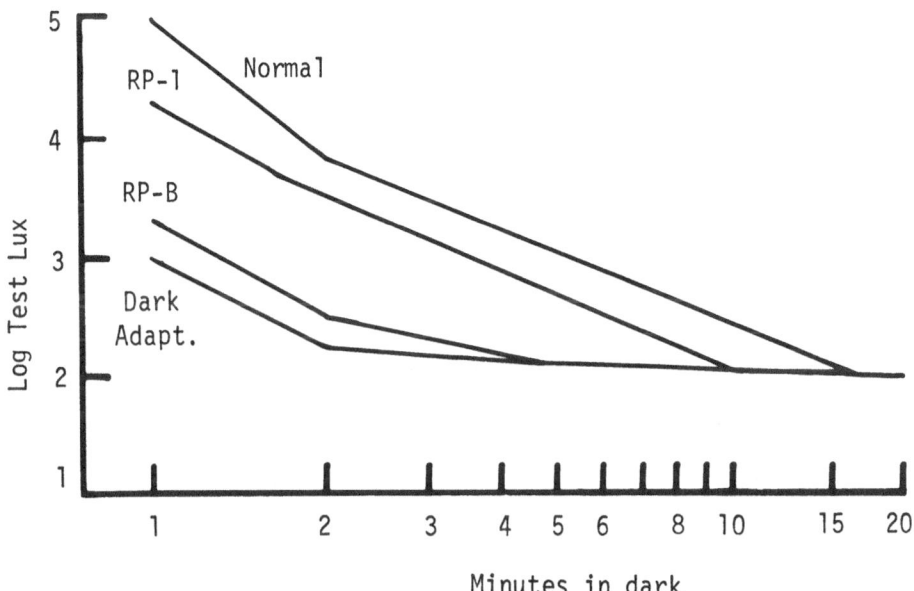

FIGURE 2. The effects of various filters on dark adaptation. RP-1 and RP-B are amber and bronze filter spectacles, respectively, from Glendale Optical Company. Dark adapt is a commercial dark adaptation filter (American Cyanamid Red R8613-80). The absorption curves of these filters are shown in Fig. 1. All dark adaptation curves are averaged from three runs on a Goldmann adaptometer (Haag–Streit Model 395). There was no preadaptation bleach and each filter was worn approximately one half hour binocularly in the normal lights in the laboratory rooms.

whose phosphor has its maximum output at not less than 580 nm. It should have as little emission as possible at shorter wavelengths than this. Possibly a phosphor which peaks at about 600 nm would be of maximum use.

The ophthalmic examination itself should minimize exposure to unfiltered light. Bleaching lights in any procedures such as the electroretinogram (ERG), the electrooculogram (EOG) and dark adaptation should be minimized by combining the procedures whenever possible or by eliminating them entirely. The same caution should be exercized in the use of high intensity stimulus presentations.

Elevation of Retinal Temperature

There are many indications that an elevated retinal temperature or body temperature renders the eye more susceptible to damage
by high light intensity such as is typical of laser exposure (Ward
and Bruce, 1971). This is also true of retinal dystrophy in rats
(Noell *et al.*, 1966), although at much lower light and temperature
levels, and is presumably also true in retinitis pigmentosa. These
elevated body temperatures are well within the physiological range.
It would seem indicated to avoid light during any fever and to act
aggressively with the appropriate drugs to reduce any acute temperature rise. Perhaps a lower than normal body temperature on a
chronic basis would inhibit the course of degeneration in retinitis
pigmentosa. However, there is no experimental data in this direction. Examination of patients who take chlorpromazine or morphine
on a regular basis might furnish guidance in this matter. It
has been suggested that male and female siblings might exhibit
different disease courses about puberty, with the elevated body
temperatures associated with menstruation accelerating the disease
in women but not in men (H. Delleman, personal communication,
1974). The relevant records are now under examination.

It should be noted that infrared admitted into the eye along
with the visible light will raise the retinal temperature without
contributing significantly to vision. To eliminate this effect all
spectacles should have an infrared filter, especially when used in
sunlight. An absorption curve for a filter incorporating this
feature (Glendale RP-B) is shown in Fig. 1.

A similar constraint should be applied also to the instruments used in ophthalmic examinations. Although most ophthalmic
instruments already have infrared absorbing filters in them, the
efficiency of these in most cases can be considerably improved.
Table I shows the proportion of the total radiation removed from a
fundus camera and indirect ophthalmoscope by the insertion of an
infrared filter. The use of tungsten-halogen lamps for illumination increases the problem. Although these lamps have a higher
color temperature with a correspondingly higher proportion of the
radiation in the visible than usual lamps, the increased total
output still has a higher absolute level of infrared than the
regular tungsten bulb.

Vitamin A and Other Metabolic Factors

There are several indications that normal rod function is
quite dependent upon the level of vitamin A. The continued growth
of the outer segment depends upon the easy availability of vitamin
A. As has been mentioned earlier, one of the first symptoms of
vitamin A deficiency is inhibition of rod function accompanied by

TABLE I

EFFECT OF INFRARED FILTER ON ENERGY OUTPUT
MEASURED IN MICROWATTS/CM^2 AT APPROXIMATE POSITION OF PUPIL

	Zeiss Fundus Flash Lamp	Camera Focus Lamp	AO Indirect Ophthalmoscope (brightest setting)
Normal	6.1	5.5	5
With IR filter	4.0	3.5	3.5

The addition of an infrared filter to each of these instruments results in a reduction of nearly one third in the corneal energy.

disappearance of the outer segment. Noell and Albrecht (1971)
have shown that vitamin A deficiency protects against light induced
degeneration of the retina. Herron and Riegel (1974) have shown
that vitamin A levels low enough to inhibit rod outer segment formation apparently have little effect on the cones in normal rats,
at least for a short time. However, clinically it is difficult
to attain marked total vitamin A deficiency without other side
effects. Vitamin A supplements have been suggested as a symptomatic treatment for retinitis pigmentosa, specifically to alleviate
the symptoms of night blindness and loss of peripheral vision which
retinitis pigmentosa has in common with vitamin A deficiency
(Chatzinoff et al., 1968; Bergsma and Wolf, 1975). However, this
symptomatic treatment may, in fact, be contraindicated.

In the Bassen-Kornzweig syndrome there is a failure to
metabolize some types of lipoprotein. This has led to applying
the term abetalipoproteinemia to this syndrome. Gouras et al.
(1971) have shown that the visual symptoms of this syndrome respond
well to massive doses of vitamin A, with cone function returning
before rod function. However, this particular syndrome is accompanied by blood abnormalities--muscular atrophy, neuropathy, fat
intolerances, etc. It can easily be distinguished from the classi-
cal type of retinitis pigmentosa in which there are no errors in
fat metabolism. It is thus quite important to distinguish between
the different types of retinal degeneration. A diet with supple-
mentary vitamin A would be proper therapy for the Bassen-Kornzweig
syndrome. On the other hand, typical retinitis pigmentosa cases
should perhaps have the vitamin A level kept at as low a level as
is compatible with general body health.

Rod outer segment formation can also be inhibited by restricting the essential fatty acids which are a major component of it (Landis *et al*., 1973). The same effect can be brought about by poisoning the mitochondria which are found in such high concentrations in the rod inner segment. A typical mitochondrial poison, iodoacetic acid, will selectively kill rods, while sparing the cones (Noell, 1952). These techniques offer an insight into other ways of controlling retinitis pigmentosa. However, until more is known about the long term survival of cones in the retina following such wholesale rod destruction, such avenues of therapy as these will not be ready for clinical trials.

THERAPEUTIC APPROACH

The rationale for the proposed therapy is detailed above and is based on the hypothesis that retinitis pigmentosa is a disease connected with rod activity, with the cones involved only secondarily. From this, it seems reasonable to try an experimental therapy for retinitis pigmentosa, incorporating the following points.

1. Minimize the amount of light stimulating the rods. Figure 1 shows the absorption spectrum for the spectacle lenses that we have selected. The absorption spectrum is matched closely to the absorption spectrum of rhodopsin, the rod photopigment. As the spectacles absorb heavily in the blue and green, but transmit freely from 570 nm onward, they appear yellow. Opaque or filter shields should be used around the spectacles on the sides and tops to minimize the amount of nonfiltered light reaching the eye. A photochromic glass which has a similar absorption would be very useful if such were available. The ophthalmic examination should minimize exposure to unfiltered and high intensity light.

2. Monitor the patient's temperature closely (especially in children) to detect any acute elevation from normal. An aggressive regime of appropriate drug therapy to prevent or minimize acute fevers is necessary. Properly, the patient should be kept in the dark during any fever because of the deleterious interaction of light and elevated temperature.

3. Minimize the amount of infrared radiation reaching the retina. The filter spectacles should contain an infrared filter. We have incorporated one in our filter, RP-B, as shown in Fig. 1. Also, all ophthalmic instruments should be modified to prevent as much infrared as possible from entering the patient's eye.

4. Minimize vitamin A intake and body levels. Avoid vitamin supplements and foods containing large amounts of vitamin A. In view of the fact that vitamin A supplements have often been

proposed for therapy, it seems that at the very least a warning is in order to prevent high doses of vitamin A as a symptomatic treatment for the night blindness associated with retinitis pigmentosa.

ASSESSMENT OF EFFICACY OF TREATMENT AND SUGGESTIONS FOR FUTURE RESEARCH

The assessment of the efficacy of the treatment can only be based upon the assumption that family members will have a similar, although not identical, time course of the disease. Thus, cases can only be selected for assessment where there are other family members who have well documented time courses for the disease. Only in this way can it be possible to assess whether a patient on this therapeutic regime has the expected course of his disease modified. Although no formal conclusion could be drawn from a single record, the evaluation of a considerable number of cases should show whether any definite change could be attributed to this therapeutic regime.

More research is needed before we would advocate the substitution of vitamin A acid for vitamin A in the diet and the administration of metabolic (particularly mitochondrial) inhibitors, such as iodoacetic acid, which Noell (1952) has shown to inhibit rod function or cause rod (but not cone) degeneration. New therapeutic filters and new animal models are needed, but most of all a better diagnosis and documentation of the particular disease process of each patient and his family members. To accomplish this end, there is a need for clinical tests which are both more subtle and more objective.

ACKNOWLEDGEMENTS

We are grateful for the technical assistance of our colleagues Mr. M. Bessler, Dr. B. Yamanashi, and Ms. M. A. Orr. Dr. Werner Noell has kindly made available to us much data supplemental to his published material, and has given us many suggestions on possible interpretations of the voluminous literature.

Portions of this work have been presented at the 1974 Annual Meeting of the Association for Research in Vision and Ophthalmology in a report by M. L. Wolbarsht and M. B. Landers, III entitled "Control of Retinitis Pigmentosa by Inhibition of Rod Outer Segment Growth from Vitamin A Deficiency or Metabolic Poisons."

Portions of this research were supported by a grant from the North Carolina Association for the Blind, Inc.

REFERENCES

Anderson, B., Jr. (1968) Ocular effects of changes in oxygen and carbon dioxide tension. *Trans. Amer. Ophthal. Soc.* 66:423.

Bennett, M. H., Dyer, R. F., and Dunn, J. D. (1973) Visual deficit following long term continuous light exposure. *Exper. Neurol.* 38:80.

Bergsma, D. R. and Wolf, M. L. (1977) A therapeutic trial of vitamin A in patients with pigmentary retinal degenerations: a negative study, in "Retinitis Pigmentosa: Clinical Implications of Current Research" (M. B. Landers, M. L. Wolbarsht, J. E. Dowling, and A. M. Laties, eds.) pp. 197-209, Plenum Press, New York.

Berson, E. L. (1971) Light deprivation for early retinitis pigmentosa. *Arch. Ophthal.* 85:521.

Berson, E. L. and Howard, J. (1971) Temporal aspects of the electroretinogram in sector retinitis pigmentosa. *Arch. Ophthal.* 86:653-665.

Berson, E. L., Rabin, A. R., and MeHaffey, L. (1973) Advances in night vision technology. *Arch. Ophthal.* 90:427.

Char, D. H., Bergsma, D. R., Rabson, A. S., Albert, D. M., and Herberman, R. B. (1974) Cell-mediated immunity to retinal antigens in patients with pigmentary retinal degenerations. *Invest. Ophthal.* 13:198.

Chatzinoff, A., Nelson, E., Stahl, N., and Clahane, A. (1968) Eleven-cis vitamin A in the treatment of retinitis pigmentosa. *Arch. Ophthal.* 80:417-419.

Dowling, J. E. and Wald, G. (1960) The role of vitamin A acid. *Vitamins and Hormones* 18:515.

Dowling, J. E. and Gibbons, I. R. (1961) The effect of vitamin A deficiency on the fine structure of the retina, in "Structure of the Eye" (G. K. Smelser, ed.) pp. 85-99, Academic Press, New York.

Feeney, L. (1973) The phagolysosomal system of the pigment epithelium. A key to retinal disease. *Arch. Ophthal.* 12:635.

Gorn, R. A. and Kuwabara, T. (1967) Retinal damage by visible light, a physiological study. *Arch. Ophthal.* 77:115.

Gouras, P., Carr, R. E., and Gunkel, R. D. (1971) Retinitis pigmentosa in abetalipoproteinemia: effects of vitamin A. *Invest. Ophthal.* 10:784.

Herron, W. L., Jr. and Riegel, B. W. (1974) Vitamin A deficiency-induced "rod thinning" to permanently decrease the production of rod outer segment material. *Invest. Ophthal.* 13:54.

Herron, W. L., Jr., Riegel, B. W., Brennan, E., and Rubin, M. L. (1974) Retinal dystrophy in the pigmented rat. *Invest. Ophthal.* 13:87.

Kolb, H. and Gouras, P. (1974) Electron microscopic observations of human retinitis pigmentosa, dominantly inherited. *Invest. Ophthal.* 13:487.

Landis, D. J., Dudley, P. A., and Anderson, R. E. (1973) Alteration of disc formation in photoreceptors of rat retina. *Science* 182:1144.

Lawwill, T. (1973) Effects of prolonged exposure of rabbit retina to low-intensity light. *Invest. Ophthal.* 12:45.

Noell, W. K. (1952) The impairment of visual cell structure by iodoacetate. *J. Cell. Comp. Physiol.* 40:25.

Noell, W. K., Walker, V. S., Kang, B. S., and Berman, S. (1966) Retinal damage by light in rats. *Invest. Ophthal.* 5:450.

Noell, W. K. and Albrecht, R. (1971) Irreversible effects of visible light on the retina: role of vitamin A. *Science* 172:76-80.

O'Steen, W. K. and Anderson, K. V. (1971) Photically evoked responses in the visual system of rats exposed to continuous light. *Exp. Neurol.* 30:525.

Tso, M. O. M. (1973) Photic maculopathy in rhesus monkey. *Invest. Ophthal.* 12:17.

Ward, B. and Bruce, W. R. (1971) Chorioretinal burn: body temperature dependence. *Ann. Ophthal.* 3:898.

Young, R. W. (1973) Renewal systems in rods and cones. *Ann. Ophthal.* 5:843.

DISCUSSION OF THE PAPER

DR. LAVAIL: In animals that are kept in the dark or those
with pigmented eyes, you do have a slowing down of the disease, but
at the same time, you actually have a thicker debris zone earlier
on than you do in the pink-eyed animals. So it is just sort of the
inverse of what you would intuitively feel based on your hypothesis.

DR. LANDERS: Myron, do you have a comment?

DR. WOLBARSHT: Well, there are a lot of questions. The three
published cases were so old at the time of death that it was difficult to say what the disease was. It would be hard to see debris
even in the rats of comparable age. This is long after the whole
retina has disappeared. I would really say that retinitis pigmentosa is an open matter just because we don't have the pathology.
All of your comments are quite relevant, and in fact quite realis-
tic. Still all we can say is that this is a model that we can look
at now and think about. Certainly the first problem is that retinitis pigmentosa certainly is not a single disease. What is true
of one form may not be true of another form. At the moment we
can't distinguish between them.

DR. LEWIS: Are there any commercially available glasses that
are suitable for helping cases of retinitis pigmentosa, or is anything being done along that line?

DR. LANDERS: The answer is a hopeful "no." There are glasses
available. Wolbarsht and I have been working on glasses; we have
some suitable ones. If you get into the glasses business, the next
thing you know is that you have a lot of people calling you. They
may have retinitis pigmentosa, or they may have senile macular
degeneration, cancer of the eye, and so on. We are really not
advocating that people start putting glasses on patients on the
basis of what we are saying. We have a model. There is an old
saying "better to light one candle than curse the darkness." I
don't know if the model is right. Obviously people are not rats,
but it is a start. If you have a retinitis pigmentosa clinic,
you find that you will take anything as a start. We are very
concerned, though, that word not go around that everybody with
retinitis pigmentosa should rush out and purchase some amber
colored glasses. I think that is a real mistake. I think that
this possibly should be tried in a controlled situation, a controlled environment. However, just to do control studies on
patients whose disease lasts as long as the life of the investigator is very, very difficult. So, I want to say "no" there aren't
glasses. If you shop around you can find various companies making
these colored glasses, but I think that at this stage that is a

mistake and it might even confuse some findings which could be obtained from a controlled study.

DR. LEWIS: Should you ask a patient who has retinitis pigmentosa to wear any kind of dark glasses in the bright sunlight?

DR. LANDERS: Well, I wear them. I'm not against that. It is one thing to say that theoretically it might be good; it is quite another to tell a patient that you are treating him or that he is treating himself when he does this.

DR. SANDBERG: There has been a lot of talk at these meetings about the relevance and relationship of vitamin A and RP and I just wanted to say—and this is strictly preliminary. We have traced the recovery of a patient with a vitamin A deficiency from practically total blindness to normality after we have been giving him pretty large doses. I wanted to comment that both in terms of the ERG and in terms of some of my psychophysical testing, his condition looked very, very much different from RP. It is very easy to separate the two in terms of relative rod and cone impairment in different retinal areas. I depended very much on retinal area. The cones did get very much impaired. They were very photophobic.

Another, more theoretical, note. If you do decide to decrease vitamin A in these patients, you should keep in mind that, as has been shown many times before in basic research, there is a very dramatic threshold elevation just from decreasing vitamin A in the retina, a logarithmic relationship. It is like cutting off the neck to cure a cold.

A THERAPEUTIC TRIAL OF VITAMIN A IN PATIENTS WITH PIGMENTARY

RETINAL DEGENERATIONS: A NEGATIVE STUDY

Donald R. Bergsma and Mitchel L. Wolf*

Clinical Branch, National Eye Institute
National Institutes of Health
Bethesda, Maryland 20014

The Jewish Hospital of St. Louis*
Department of Ophthalmology
Washington University School of Medicine
660 South Euclid Avenue
St. Louis, Missouri 63110

INTRODUCTION

Retinitis pigmentosa and other pigmentary retinal degenerations have defied effective therapy since their identification a
century ago, shortly after the discovery of the ophthalmoscope.

Although the striking similarities between the visual loss of
retinitis pigmentosa and that of dietary induced vitamin A deficiency are well known, no convincing evidence has been published
to indicate that vitamin A therapy is usually successful in
patients suffering from retinitis pigmentosa. Because these
diseases are generally only slowly progressive and involve functions such as side vision and dark adaptation which the patient
cannot measure accurately, it is not surprising that patients
could become convinced that improvement had occurred following
ineffective treatment. Moreover, even when performed in a medical
setting, such measurements are subject to learning effect, motivation, and other variations.

Indirect and sometimes contradictory evidence is available
from serum measurements of vitamin A (retinol) and retinol-binding
protein. Campbell and Tonks (1962) found that the average vitamin
A concentration was lower than normal in sera of patients with
retinitis pigmentosa. This was not found to be true in a more

recent study by Futterman *et al.* (1974). Similarly, Rahi (1972) reported low serum retinol-binding protein (RBP) levels in patients with retinitis pigmentosa, but a more recent study by Maraini *et al.* (1975) found no difference from normal in a small group of patients with different genetic types of retinitis pigmentosa.

Likewise, therapeutic trials of vitamin A administered to patients with retinitis pigmentosa have produced inconclusive results. Gordon (1948), in a study involving 128 patients, concluded that the apparent improvement which some of his patients had demonstrated after treatment with cod liver oil, vitamin A, or placental implant (the "Filatov method") might have been due to factors other than organic improvement such as learning effect, testing scatter, and motivation; thus the issue was left unresolved. In 1964, Campbell *et al.* published a preliminary report of a controlled therapeutic trial of treatment of retinitis pigmentosa patients with vitamin A and E. Their studies suggested greater improvement of visual field and cone function with vitamin A and E than with vitamin A alone. Unfortunately, to the best of my knowledge the results of the completed study were never published. Chatzinoff *et al.* (1968) published negative results using 11-cis vitamin A in the treatment of retinitis pigmentosa. Later Chatzinoff (1969), in a letter to the editor, mentioned improvement in a 10 year old patient given 11-cis vitamin A, but regression in the sibling who was given a trial of all-trans vitamin A. Gouras *et al.* (1971) demonstrated that massive oral doses (200,000 I.U.) of all-trans vitamin A palmitate produced repeated acute and prolonged improvement of both electroretinographic and psychophysical responses in two patients with abetalipoproteinemia (Bassen-Kornzweig disease). Unfortunately, the long term downhill course of these patients over a period of years was not stopped by vitamin A administration (personal observation).

I will make no attempt to review the extensive and important work on vitamin A deprivation and therapy in animals and in animal models of retinal dystrophy. Nevertheless, the reader should be alerted that the situation is complex. In two recent studies Herron and Riegel (1974a, 1974b) suggested that vitamin A deficiency (*not excess*) might be beneficial in certain types of retinal dystrophy because it reduces the production rate of rod outer segment material which builds up in retinal dystrophic rats. These papers will also lead the reader to relevant animal studies performed by Dowling, by Kuwabara, by LaVail, by Noell, and by Young, all of whom are making other contributions to this symposium.

Because the effectiveness of vitamin A in treating retinitis pigmentosa was left unresolved by the above evidence, a prospective therapeutic trial of high dosage vitamin A therapy for pigmentary retinal degenerations was undertaken with emphasis on obtaining multiple parameters of visual function on two separate occasions prior to the administration of vitamin A.

MATERIALS AND METHODS

A prospective study was designed to test the hypothesis that high dosages of vitamin A might produce measurable visual improvement in some patients with pigmentary retinal degenerations. Patients were drawn from the retinal degeneration clinic at the National Eye Institute. For a period of six months all new and return patients with pigmentary retinal degenerations who were not recently nor currently taking high doses of vitamin A on their own were given an explanation of the trial and an opportunity to participate. Multivitamins containing 5,000 international units of vitamin A were considered low dosage and, therefore, not a contraindication to participation. These patients had already had an initial workup consisting of general ophthalmic examinations, visual fields performed on the Goldmann perimeter, color vision testing using Hardy Rand-Rittler pseudoisochromatic plates, Farnsworth Panel D-15 (and when indicated the Nagel anomaloscope), dark adaptation using the Goldmann-Weekers dark adaptometer, cone threshold measurements as described by Gunkel (1967), fundus photography, and electroretinography as described by Gouras (1970), Rabin and Berson (1974), and Gunkel et al. (1976). Blood was drawn for vitamin A determination and other analyses at each visit. Table I summarizes the protocol for the first visit. A summary of the protocol for the second visit is presented in Table II. The second visit consisted of measurements of visual acuity, visual

TABLE I

PROTOCOL FOR FIRST VISIT

I.   OCULAR AND GENERAL HISTORY
     (emphasis on family history and drug history)

II. GENERAL OCULAR EXAMINATION
     --Fields (kinetic on Goldmann Perimeter)
     --Dark adaptation and cone thresholds
     --Color vision (D-15, HRR, ±anomaloscope)
     --Fundus photography
     --Electroretinography

III. STANDARD LABS, SEROLOGY, VITAMIN A, CAROTENE

fields, color vision, dark adaptation, and cone thresholds to obtain a second set of pretrial data on each patient. A few tests
which differed significantly from the first visit were repeated an
extra time on the second visit. The therapeutic trial consisted of
50,000 I.U. of water-solubilized vitamin A [Aquasol (R) A Capsules
50,000 I.U., U S V Pharmaceutical Corporation, New York, New York;
Composition: all-trans vitamin A_1 (retinol) water-solubilized
using sorethytan oleate esters] orally per day for 28 days. The
single child in the study received 50,000 I.U. every other day.
The protocol for the third visit is summarized in Table III. The
third visit occurred at the end of four weeks on vitamin A and
included all the tests listed for the second pretrial visit.
Patients were instructed to call immediately to arrange for early
testing if their vision changed noticeably after starting the
therapeutic trial. Post-trial electroretinography was performed
only on 10 patients selected by the authors from among the patients
who had a recordable pre-trial electroretinogram. Ten patients
(four patients with unusual immediate post-trial results and six
others from among those living close by) have returned at six month
and one year intervals, others have not reached these landmarks or
are on longer follow-up intervals. One patient was withdrawn from
the study after two weeks because of headaches. No attempt was
made to mask the study for the following reasons. First, the
emphasis was on careful, repeated testing of multiple functions in
a variety of pigmentary retinal degenerations. Therefore, assuming
that we were dealing with a heterogeneous group of diseases in
which only an unknown proportion might respond to the therapy being
tested, it was determined that the effort would be too great to

TABLE II

PROTOCOL FOR SECOND VISIT

ESTABLISH SEPARATE PRE-TRIAL MEASUREMENTS:

    --Visual acuity
    --Fields
    --Dark adaptation and cone thresholds
    --Color vision
    --Vitamin A, carotene (electroretinography,
        if first results unsatisfactory)

    (NOTE: Patients were instructed to return
            immediately if their vision changed
            subjectively on therapy.)

reach statistically significant results if half the patients were placed on placebo medication. Second, since vitamin A in the dosage we were using has a unique capsule, no placebo was readily available. Third, it was our intention, if successful therapeutic results were obtained on a prospective study, to invest the additional effort which would be required for a randomized masked study, whereas negative results would indicate that this effort is unnecessary.

In discussing the therapeutic trial with the patients, the ophthalmologists attempted to convey their dedication to the necessity of determining whether or not vitamin A therapy is useful for pigmentary retinal degenerations because other studies had been inconclusive. Moreover, the estimated probability of the vitamin A trial producing improvement of the participants' vision was stated to be low but not precisely definable. Perhaps because of the low risk involved and a desire to find hope somewhere, the overwhelming majority of patients given the opportunity to participate decided to do so. Moreover, of the 48 patients entered into the study, all but the one who was removed because of headaches returned for the second pre-trial and the post-trial examinations. Several postponements of the second pre-trial visit occurred, but all post-trial appointments occurred as scheduled with the minor exception that three patients' doses were continued to 35 days before the post-trial examination occurred instead of the planned 28 days.

TABLE III

PROTOCOL FOR THIRD VISIT

MEASUREMENTS AFTER 28 DAYS THERAPEUTIC TRIAL OF
AQUASOL A, 50,000 I.U. po DAILY

--Visual acuity
--Fields
--Dark adaptation and cone thresholds
--Color vision
--Vitamin A and carotene
  (Electroretinography on 10 selected patients)

(Note: A subset of 10 patients was seen one
       month and six months later for repeat
       measurements.)

TABLE IV

DIAGNOSTIC CATEGORIES OF PATIENTS
TREATED WITH VITAMIN A

Retinitis pigmentosa (sporadic or recessive)	21
Retinitis pigmentosa (autosomal dominant)	6
Retinitis pigmentosa and deafness	5
Atypical retinitis pigmentosa	6
Cone-rod degeneration	2
Toxic retinopathy (chloroquine, thioridazine)	2
Juvenile macular degeneration	3
Choroideremia	2
TOTAL	47

Initially all patients seen with pigmentary retinal degenerations were entered into the study. Near the end of the study the
first author stopped entering patients with autosomal recessive
or sporadic retinitis pigmentosa but continued entering more unusual cases such as autosomal dominant retinitis pigmentosa, fundus
flavimaculatus and cone-rod degeneration in an attempt to test the
effect of vitamin A on a larger number of independent disease categories. The concentration of patients with the Usher syndrome
occurred early in the study because several patients had been
referred from a college for the deaf. The diagnostic categories of
patients treated with vitamin A in this study are presented in
Table IV. Their ages are presented in Table V.

The patients who participated in this study are being re-
examined at long intervals. None of the patients were continued on
vitamin A after the initial therapeutic trial.

RESULTS

The results of this therapeutic trial are summarized in Table
VI. The average serum vitamin A concentration rose from mid normal
range to high normal range (normal range 65-250 I.U. per 100 ml).
Fifteen patients achieved supernormal levels. The data strongly
indicate that a four week course of solubilized vitamin A given
orally in high dosages to patients with retinitis pigmentosa and
other pigmentary retinal degenerations does not produce measurable
improvement of visual function. Of the 47 patients tested, none
felt strongly enough that their vision had improved on therapy to
make arrangements for an early appointment as suggested, although

TABLE V

AGES OF PATIENTS TREATED WITH VITAMIN A

Age in Years	Number of Patients
10	1
14-20	11
21-30	13
31-40	7
41-50	8
51-60	4
61-68	3
TOTAL	47

several reported that they might have experienced a small amount of improvement seeing in poor light. Most were emphatic that there was no noticeable difference on therapy. Three patients had isolated tests which might suggest significant improvement after therapy. Of these, one patient had improvement of four lines on visual acuity testing in one eye. This eye, however, was amblyopic secondary to esotropia and perhaps was not measured to its best visual acuity initially. Another patient had recorded improvement of two lines on visual acuity testing in both eyes, but she continued to make errors over two lines so the end points were not precise. Finally, one patient produced what appeared to be improvement of the visual field in each eye in the mid periphery and periphery. Because of this possible improvement, the fields were retested by the initial perimetrist and by the first author on that day and two subsequent occasions and were found to be variable and borderline in the areas which appeared to have improved on the first post-trial testing session. The 10 year old girl with autosomal dominantly inherited retinitis pigmentosa was not among those with any improvement. No significant change in visual function was detected in the 10 patients retested at six month and one year intervals after the therapeutic trial. This group includes the four patients with visual acuity or visual field changes on the immediate post-trial examination detailed above. None of the patients have been given vitamin A since the original one month trial. No patients showed significant loss of visual function during the short interval in which their trial occurred.

TABLE VI

RESULTS ON 47 PATIENTS

--No significant change in dark adaptation, cone thresholds,
    color vision, or ERG
--1 patient with possibly significant improvement of visual
    fields OU
--1 patient with 2 line improvement of visual acuity OU
--1 patient with 4 line improvement of visual acuity, one
    eye (esotropia)
--No patient with striking subjective improvement
--No patient with significant improvement on more than one
    parameter

DISCUSSION

Because there was no overall improvement of the group on
therapy and no improvement in any individual which was greater than
within the limits of test reproducibility (with the possible exception of the visual acuity in the amblyopic eye) we conclude that if
visual improvement does occur in adult patients with pigmentary
retinopathy treated with high doses of vitamin A, it must either
be a rare occurrence in the common forms of retinitis pigmentosa
or in a rare type (such as that caused by abetalipoproteinemia)
which we have missed on a statistical sampling basis. Tables VII
and VIII present examples of confidence limits for the hypothetical
situation in which 40 events are measured in a homogeneous binomial
population. Because the group is heterogeneous it is not possible
to give exact confidence limits on the percentage of successful
responders to vitamin A therapy which could exist in the world of
pigmentary retinal degenerations and still be missed in a study
of this size. Still one can conclude that if they exist the number
is small and that rather than attempting large and costly studies
to screen for such exceptional hypothetical cases, the burden of
proof should rest on intensive study of individual patients in whom
there is some reason to suspect that vitamin A therapy has been or
would be of value.

The negative results of vitamin A therapy should not be interpreted as negating an important role of vitamin A in pigmentary
retinal degenerations. The studies presented in the introduction
attest to its importance in certain circumstances. The possibility
still exists of a local retinal or pigment epithelial defect in
vitamin A metabolism as suggested by Cogan (1950) and by Zeavin and

TABLE VII

CONFIDENCE LIMITS

In sampling from a binomial population with the proportion of a specified event occurring designated p, and a sample of size $n = 40$, then confidence limits for p based on the number of observed occurrences X are:

| | Confidence Limits | |
Observed	95%	99%
X = 0 out of 40	(0, 0.09)	(0, 0.12)
X = 1 out of 40	(0.0006, 0.13)	(0.0001, 0.17)

Wald (1956). More importantly, the complexity of the transport and function of vitamin A and related compounds in the various tissues, particularly the eye, is currently being explored by methods which identify and characterize vitamin A (retinol) receptors in various tissue components, especially in the cytosol fraction. Further information about vitamin A (retinol) receptors and its function is available in an editorial by Gouras and Chader (1974) and in the proceedings of a recent symposium on the pigment epithelium and retina, edited by O'Brien (1976).

SUMMARY

A prospective therapeutic trial was designed to test the hypothesis that measurable improvement of retinal functions might occur in some patients with pigmentary retinal degeneration when placed on high doses of solubilized vitamin A (Aquasol A, 50,000 I.U. per day by mouth for 28 days). After a standard ophthalmic history and examination pre-trial examinations consisting of visual acuity, visual fields, color vision tests, dark adaptations and cone thresholds were obtained on two separate occasions. Electroretinography was usually performed only once.

Forty-seven patients were entered into the study of which 27 had typical retinitis pigmentosa. The patients showed no significant change in visual function from pre-trial results when tested

TABLE VIII

CONFIDENCE LIMITS AFTER 0 OUT OF 40
RESPONSES TO TREATMENT

--95% confidence that the proportion of responders
    actually lies between 0 and 9%
--99% confidence that the proportion of responders
    actually lies between 0 and 17%
(In a negative study, the number of samples needed
 to reduce the projected proportion of responders
 towards zero rises astronomically.)

after taking the vitamin A for 28 days.   Post-trial electroretinography performed on 10 patients with recordable pre-trial electroretinograms showed no change. The 10 patients retested at six and
12 months after the trial showed no significant change in visual
function.

ACKNOWLEDGEMENTS

    The authors wish to thank Ralph Gunkel, O.D., for his advice
and performance of color vision, cone threshold, and dark adaptation measurements, to thank Miss Mary Hendricks for performing
visual fields and electrophysiologic measurements, and to thank
Roy Milton, Ph.D., for his advice and help with statistical evaluation of the results.

REFERENCES

Campbell, D. A., Harrison, R., and Tonks, E. L. (1964) Retinitis
    pigmentosa: vitamin A serum levels in relation to clinical
    findings. *Exp. Eye Res*. 3:412.

Campbell, D. A., and Tonks, E. L. (1962)   Biochemical findings in
    human retinitis pigmentosa with particular relation to vitamin
    A deficiency. *Brit. J. Ophthal*. 46:151.

Chatzinoff, A. (1969) Letter to the Editor. *Arch. Ophthal*. 82:295.

Chatzinoff, A., Nelson, E., Stahl, N., and Clahane, M. S. (1968)
    Eleven-cis vitamin A in the treatment of retinitis pigmentosa.
    A negative study. *Arch. Ophthal*. 80:417.

Cogan, D. (1950) Primary chorioretinal aberrations with night blindness. *Trans. Amer. Acad. Ophthalmol.* 54:629.

Futterman, S., Swanson, D., and Kalina, R. E. (1974) Retinol in retinitis pigmentosa: Evidence that retinol is in normal concentration in serum and the retinal-binding protein complex displays unaltered fluorescence properties. *Invest. Ophthal.* 13:798.

Gordon, D. M. (1948) The experimental treatment of retinitis pigmentosa. *Trans. Amer. Acad. Ophthal. Otolaryn.* 52:191.

Gouras, P. (1970) Electroretinography, some basic principles. *Invest. Ophthal.* 9:557.

Gouras, P., Carr, R. E., and Gunkel, R. D. (1971) Retinitis pigmentosa in abetalipoproteinemia: effects of vitamin A. *Invest. Ophthal.* 10:784.

Gouras, P., and Chader, G. (1974) Retinitis pigmentosa and retinol-binding protein (editorial). *Invest. Ophthal.* 13:239

Gunkel, R. D. (1967) Retinal profiles. *Arch. Ophthal.* 77:22.

Gunkel, R. D., Bergsma, D. R., and Gouras, P. (1976) A ganzfeld stimulator for electroretinography. *Arch. Ophthal.* 94:669.

Herron, W. L., Jr., and Riegel, B. W. (1974a) Production rate and removal of rod outer segment material in vitamin A deficiency. *Invest. Ophthal.* 13:46.

Herron, W. L., Jr., and Riegel, B. W. (1974b) Vitamin A deficiency-induced "rod thinning" to permanently decrease the production of rod outer segment material. *Invest. Ophthal.* 13:54.

Maraini, G., Fadda, G., and Gozzoli, F. (1975) Serum levels of retinol-binding protein in different genetic types of retinitis pigmentosa. *Invest. Ophthal.* 14:236.

O'Brien, P. J. (ed.) (1976) Proceedings of the National Eye Institute Symposium on the Pigment Epithelium: Its Relationship to the Retina in Health and Disease. *Exp. Eye Res.* (Symposium Issues) Pt. I, 22(5):395; Pt. II, 23:89.

Rabin, A. R., and Berson, E. L. (1974) A full-field system for clinical electroretinography. *Arch. Ophthal.* 92:59.

Rahi, A. H. S. (1972) Retinol-binding protein (RBP) and pigmentary dystrophy of the retina. *Brit. J. Ophthal.* 56:647.

Zeavin, B. H., and Wald, G. (1956) Rod and cone vision in retinitis pigmentosa. *Amer. J. Ophthal.* 42:253.

DISCUSSION OF THE PAPER

DR. SIEGEL: I agree with you completely about not proceeding
hurriedly with vitamin A therapy, but I wonder if it might not be
downright dangerous, considering what we know now from Professor
Noell's studies on the effect of hyper vitamin A levels.

DR. BERGSMA: Well, all I can say is that (1), these patients
did not get worse, and (2), there are a lot of patients out there
taking vitamin A on their own, and I don't mean just the 5,000
units per day in multivitamins. I have been impressed that many
patients, for one reason or another--on the advice of a physician,
or by their own lights--are taking the big league pills and if they
had been taking high doses on their own they were excluded from
this study because I couldn't analyze that. But no, I didn't see
any loss of vision related to their test in this limited group of
patients.

MR. CHAITIN: In a study by Campbell and Tonks, they administered vitamin A also and found that a majority of their patients
had a dramatic improvement in visual fields.

DR. BERGSMA: I didn't see a paper of hers where she actually
administered vitamin A. The one I saw was just reporting the low
levels. (The work referred to by Mr. Chaitin was later incorporated into the text. D.R.B.)

MR. CHAITIN: Well, they did a study on the same people who
had the low vitamin A levels and I just wondered if the preparation
of vitamin A that you used might be different in some way from the
preparation that they used or either that Dr. Chatzinoff used?

DR. BERGSMA: Chatzinoff used several different ones. This
one is the one that is presumably most readily absorbed orally. I
would like to see that paper if you could give me the reference.

MR. CHAITIN: Another thing. I took part in that study that
Dr. Chatzinoff undertook when I was younger and I noticed an
improvement in the night blindness that I had over the two and one
half years that I was in that study. His conclusion was that in
their life span, some people continue to get worse and some people
stay the same. Now, if you do a study like that and you find out
that some people improve, why not try to make that serum available
to them?

DR. LATIES: I just want to ask what the relationship is between oral intake levels you are doing here and the plasma transport system.

DR. BERGSMA: Well, it is felt that the retinol-binding protein runs at a fairly high level of saturation normally, maybe 80-90%, but that when vitamin A is ingested the liver rapidly releases more aporetinol-binding protein and synthesizes it into the complete retinol-binding protein so that the level of retinol-binding protein goes up physiologically in response to increased vitamin A ingestion. Goodman and others have studied that intensively. They are internists who were more interested in the liver than the eye. The retinol-binding protein has a fairly high affinity, so that once you have any vitamin A free around, it is going to tend to bind with the retinol-binding protein and produce a high level of retinol binding. That is, there is little free vitamin A in the serum.

MR. BASTEK: Is there any consideration to giving vitamin E, the antioxidant, today along with it?

DR. BERGSMA: Well, I have thought of that. You know there are a lot of public health studies in all of the countries where they are worried about keratomalacia and every time they design one of these studies that issue comes up. I didn't give vitamin E and I don't know whether one should.

THE AMBIENT LIGHT ENVIRONMENT AND OCULAR HAZARDS

David H. Sliney

Laser Microwave Division
U.S. Army Environmental Hygiene Agency
Aberdeen Proving Ground, Maryland   21010

INTRODUCTION

It has been argued that the exposure of the retina to bright
light accelerates the retinal degeneration of retinitis pigmentosa
(Berson, 1973). This thesis has developed out of the great
increase in the study of optical hazards to the eye during the past
ten years. A gradual realization has developed that ambient levels
of exposure to ultraviolet, visible, and infrared radiation in the
environment are not an enormous factor below hazardous levels, as
was once thought. In fact, ambient levels are very close to the
borderline for creating adverse effects upon chronic exposure of
the eye. This article will review the information available
regarding the ambient levels to which the human retina is exposed
in both our natural and man-made environments. Figure 1 gives an
overview of the most common light sources and their corresponding
retinal irradiance levels (Sliney and Freasier, 1973). Irradiances
which are known to cause thermal injury to the retina within the
blink reflex (0.15-0.2 sec) are shown as a sloped line near the top
of the figure. The slope of the line represents the decrease in
retinal burn threshold with increasing image size and is predic-
table from a model of thermal injury for short exposures in the
range of approximately 0.1-1 sec. One can readily see why momentary viewing of the sun through a telescope, which increases the
sun's image size, results in a retinal burn. Most man-made
sources that are brighter than common frosted light bulbs produce
very small retinal images and one would not expect the same area of
the retina to be illuminated more than momentarily.

At retinal irradiances below approximately 0.1 W/cm^2 thermal
injury should not take place since the calculated temperature elevation in the retina is less than 1°C. It was long presumed by
many investigators that the four orders of magnitude (factor of

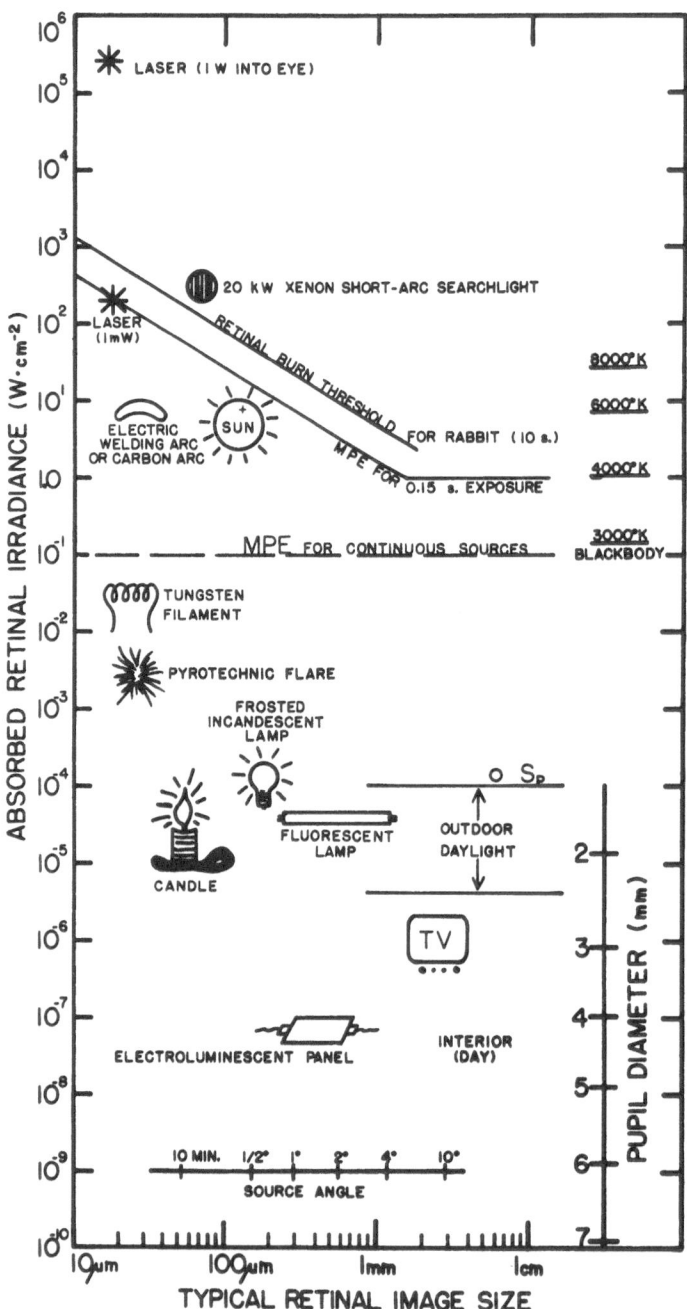

Figure 1

10,000) between thermal injury levels and most ambient levels experienced outdoors was a substantial buffer region which precluded injury from high intensity light sources, except for the sun itself, and certain very intense arc sources, or the nuclear fireball. It came as a surprise to many that light-induced retinal injury was reported in experimental animals at exposure levels of a factor of 10 to 1000 times below any thermal levels of injury (Noell and Albrecht, 1971; Kuwabara and Gorn, 1968; Harwerth and Sperling, 1975; Naidoff and Sliney, 1974; Lawwill, 1973; Ham *et al.*, 1976).

The lowest reported thresholds in primates both for functional loss determined in behavioral studies and for the production of ophthalmoscopically visible retinal lesions, occur at wavelengths in the blue region of the spectrum. These studies reported recently by Harwerth and Sperling (1975), by Ham and colleagues (1976) and by Lawwill (1973) indicate that chronic exposure to blue light at levels as low as 10^{-4} W/cm^2 in the retina causes permanent changes. Some very interesting comparisons can be made with this retinal exposure level and the environmental exposure levels of the human retina (Fig. 1).

The solar spectral radiance (brightness) for the sun at zenith has often been reported in the literature (Henderson, 1970; Robinson, 1966). The human retina is, however, seldom exposed to the direct image of the sun except at low elevation angles (Figs. 2-3). We have made measurements of the spectral radiance of sky light and of direct sunlight for a number of solar altitude angles in Maryland and California. It was noted that during clear weather the

FIGURE 1. The eye is exposed to light sources having radiances varying from $\sim 10^4$ W·cm^{-2}·sr^{-1} to $\sim 10^{-6}$ W·cm^{-2}·sr^{-1} and less. The resulting retinal irradiances vary from ~ 200 W·cm^{-2} down to 10^{-7} W·cm^{-2} and even lower; retinal irradiances are shown for typical image sizes for several sources. A minimal pupil size was assumed for intense sources, except for searchlight. The retinal burn threshold for a 10-sec exposure of the rabbit retina is shown as upper solid line. The maximum permissible exposure (MPE) applied by the U.S. Army Environmental Hygiene Agency in evaluating momentary viewing of cw light sources is shown as lower solid line. Threshold for permanent shift of blue-cone sensitivity in monkeys obtained by Sperling is shown as 0 Sp at 3×10^{-4} W·cm^{-2}. Approximate pupil sizes are shown at lower left based upon exposure of most of the retina to light of the given irradiance.

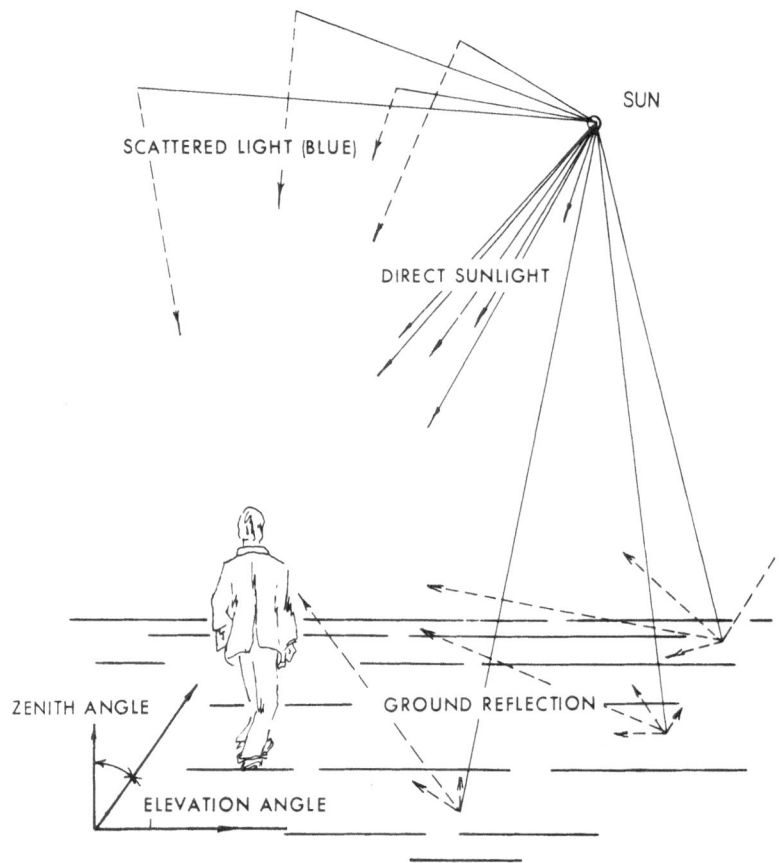

FIGURE 2. The natural light environment of man is made up of: direct sunlight, scattered light, and reflected light.

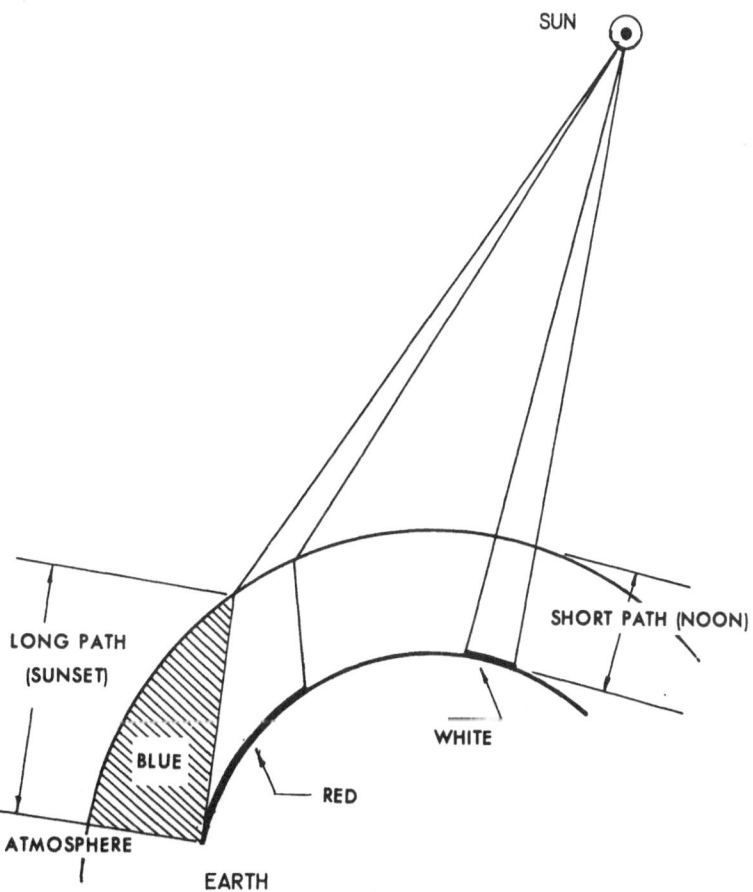

FIGURE 3. A greater fraction of the short-wavelength blue light is scattered out of the direct sunlight as sunset approaches. The refraction of sunlight by the atmosphere is exaggerated for illustration.

blue component of direct sunlight varied very little for solar elevation angles greater than 20°, the sun's position during most of
the day during summer months. In spite of the high blue component,
one seldom hears the sun described as "white"; it is usually
described as yellow or orange, with little blue. The direct solar
spectral irradiance is 1 - 1.5 W·cm^{-2}·sr^{-1}·nm at 440 nm (Fig. 4).

As sunset approaches, the relative fraction of blue light in
the direct solar spectrum dramatically decreases as the sun nears
the horizon. It was found that as long as the total solar irradiance exceeded 10 mW/cm^2, it was very difficult to look directly at
the sun and still unpleasant to have the sun imaged on the peripheral retina. However, once the total irradiance fell below
3 mW/cm^2, corresponding to an elevation angle of less than 5° in
relatively clear weather, most people found it reasonably comfortable to look at the sunset, which then lasts for only five to ten
minutes.

If a 60-nm bandwidth for this blue-light injury mechanism is
assumed, the effective blue-light irradiance on the retina for comparison with a 440-nm injury threshold can be calculated. The
retinal irradiance at 440 nm for a 60-nm spectral band is approximately 0.36 W/cm^2 at midday, and 10^{-3} to 10^{-2} W/cm^2 near sunset.
These latter values compare with the injury threshold at 441 nm of
3 x 10^{-2} W/cm^2 for 10^3 sec determined recently by Ham and his
colleagues (1976). On the other hand, the midday solar retinal
irradiance corresponds to a threshold duration of less than 100
sec. It therefore appears reasonable that the blue light damage
mechanism alone is responsible for solar retinitis.

The brightest source to which the retina can be exposed,
except for direct observation of the sun, is sunlight at noon-time
reflected from freshly fallen snow. For this source, which has a
radiance of approximately 1 mW·cm^{-2}·sr^{-1}·nm^{-1} the corresponding
retinal irradiance for a 60-nm blue light band centered at 440 nm
is 3.6 x 10^{-4} W/cm^2 for a 2-mm pupil. If one assumes that reci-
procity holds for this photochemical effect for a period of at
least eight hours, one could extrapolate that this retinal irradiance from observing snow would produce retinal injury for an
exposure duration of 8 x 10^4 sec (which is approximately 23 hours).
It is known that one aspect of snow blindness, aside from the
characteristic photokeratitis, is a substantial reduction in night
vision. Additionally, MacDonald and Fordon (1971) and others have
reported that erythropsia occurs in aphakics exposed to such bright
sources as sunlight reflected off snow. One cannot help but wonder
if the cases of prolonged erythropsia in aphakics approach a situation of permanent retinal injury. The removal of the crystalline
lens does, after all, substantially change the environment to which
the retina is exposed. Ham's recent findings (Ham *et al.*, 1976)
of a photochemical type of injury mechanism in the blue end of the

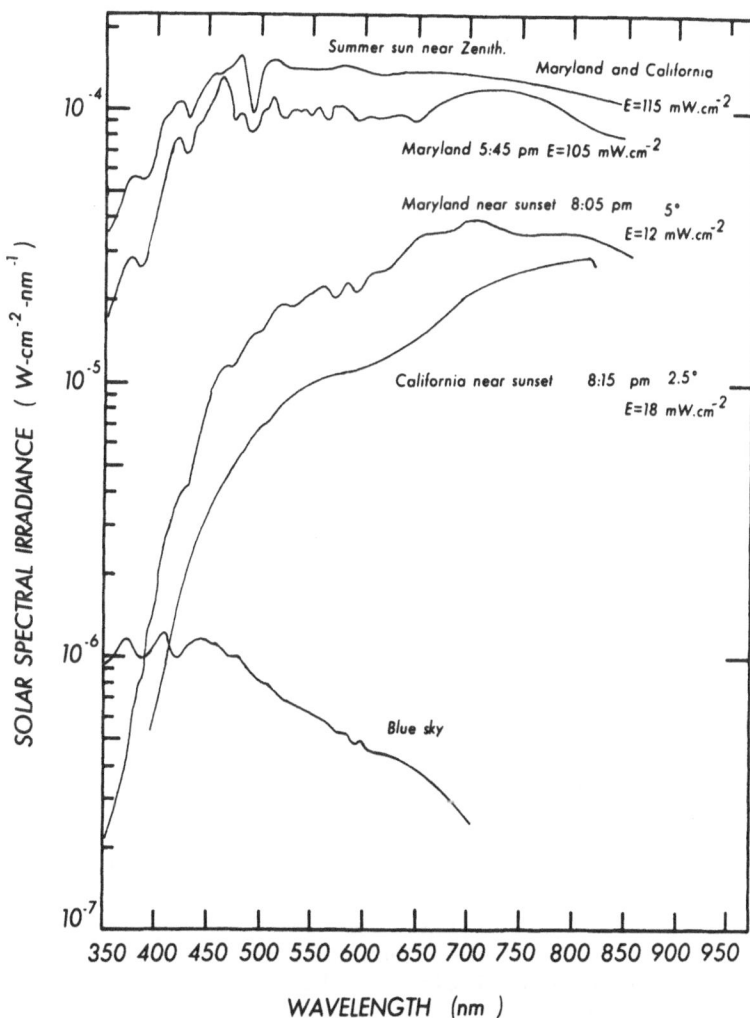

FIGURE 4. The spectral radiance of the sun is plotted for several conditions based upon measurements made near the time of summer solstice. By comparison, the spectral radiance of the blue sky (average) had to be raised three decades to be shown on the graph.

spectrum strongly suggest the need for further research on the effects of near-ultraviolet radiation which reaches the retina in aphakics. Although aphakics often receive UV-absorbing yellow spectacle lenses to reduce the adverse visual effects of chromatic aberration, these yellow lenses have not been prescribed to protect the retina from the increased exposure to ultraviolet radiation. In recent years, permanent visual functional changes have been reported in certain occupations, such as welding and foundry work (Gupta and Singh, 1968; Medvedovskaya, 1970). This once again suggests that man is adapted to his environment with very little tolerance for significant excursions in his light environment above these natural levels. During and shortly after World War II, several reports appeared which showed the reduced sensitivity of cones as well as rods in individuals exposed to desert and sea- shore environments. Permanent effects, such as those reported by Homer Smith (1944) in the U.S. Navy personnel during World War II and by Livingston (1932), also lead one to question whether there is much buffer between our natural environment and permanent changes in the retina. Although ultraviolet-induced cataractogene- sis and spheroidal degeneration of the cornea have been the subject of several epidemiologic studies (Pirie, 1972; Rodger, 1973; Fraun- felder and Hanna, 1973; Young and Finlay, 1973) it would appear that epidemiological studies of retinal changes in individuals as a function of light environment are certainly called for.

Welders given choices among various filters to use with a variety of welding arcs and gas torches selected, in almost all cases, one that reduced the luminance to approximately 1 candela per cm^2. This luminance corresponds, interestingly enough, to bright sand in full sunlight and is somewhat less than the bright- ness of sunlight reflected off snow.

To this point the discussion has been limited largely to reti- nal exposure by visible radiation. We cannot rule out the adverse effects to the retina from the very low levels of near ultraviolet radiation that reach the retina after passing through the crystal- line lens. Granted that less than 0.1% reaches the retina of the normal adult eye, this radiation could be much more effective than blue light in causing an adverse effect. Further research is clearly indicated to clarify this concern.

Any one of the observations that has been made here probably would not appear to be too striking in itself. However, taken as a whole, they support an argument that mankind is indeed adapted specifically for this environment. Any substantial alterations of the environment by man--through the use of artificial sources, through the removal of the crystalline lens of the eye, through the change of the normal spectrum of light which enters the eye--must be carefully reviewed from a standpoint of potential hazards.

REFERENCES

Berson, E. L. (1973) Experimental and therapeutic aspects of photic damage to the retina. *Invest. Ophthal.* 12:35-44.

Fraunfelder, F. T., and Hanna, C. (1973) Spheroidal degeneration of cornea and conjunctiva, 3. Incidences, classifications and etiology. *Amer. J. Ophthal.* 76:41-50.

Gupta, M. N., and Singh, H. (1968) Ocular effects and visual performance in welders. Government of India Ministry of Labour, Employment and Rehabilitation, Department of Labour and Employment, Report No. 27.

Ham, W. T., Jr., Mueller, H. A., and Sliney, D. H. (1976) Retinal sensitivity to damage from short wavelength light. *Nature* 260:153-155.

Harwerth, R. S., and Sperling, H. G. (1975) Effects of intense visible radiation on the increment-threshold spectral sensitivity of the rhesus monkey eye. *Vis. Res.* 15:1193-1204.

Henderson, S. T. (1970) "Daylight and Its Spectrum," American Elsevier, New York.

Kuwabara, T., and Gorn, R. A. (1968) Retinal damage by visible light: an electron microscopic study. *Arch. Ophthal.* 79:69.

Lawwill, T. E. (1973) Effects of prolonged exposure of rabbit retina to low-intensity light. *Invest. Ophthal.* 12:45-51.

Livingston, P. C. (1932) The study of sun glare in Iraq. *Brit. J. Ophthal.* 6:577-625.

MacDonald, J. E., and Fordon, L. (1971) Erythropsia and Light Toxicity Thresholds. Presented at the Annual Meeting of the Association for Research in Vision and Ophthalmology, Sarasota, Florida, April, 1971.

Medvedovskaya, Ts. P. (1970) Data on the condition of the eye in workers at a glass factory. *Hygiene and Sanitation* 35:445-447.

Naidoff, M. A., and Sliney, D. H. (1974) Retinal injury from a welding arc. *Amer. J. Ophthal.* 77:633.

Noell, W. K., and Albrecht, R. (1971) Irreversible effects of visible light on the retina, role of vitamin A. *Science* 172:76.

Pirie, A. (1972) The effect of sunlight on proteins of the lens, in "Contemporary Ophthalmology--Honoring Sir Stewart Duke-Elder" (J. G. Bellows, ed.) Williams and Wilkens, Baltimore.

Robinson, N. (1966) "Solar Radiation," American Elsevier, New York.

Rodgers, F. C. (1973) Clinical findings, course and progress of Biettis corneal degeneration in the Dahlak Islands. *Brit. J. Ophthal.* 57:657-661.

Sliney, D. H., and Freasier, B. C. (1973) Evaluation of optical radiation hazards. *Appl. Opt.* 12:1-22.

Smith, H. E. (1944) Actinic macular retinal pigment degeneration. *U.S. Naval Med. Bull.* 42:675-680.

Young, J. D. H., and Finlay, R. D. (1973) Primary spheroidal degeneration of the cornea in Labrador and northern Newfoundland. *Amer. J. Ophthal.* 79:129-134.

DISCUSSION OF THE PAPER

MR. CROUCH: I am very interested in this presentation. I might indicate that we approach it from a viewpoint of discomfort glare or disability glare, so our levels are much lower than anything we have been talking about here. We don't put up with bare filaments or bare fluorescent lamps--they must always be shielded and cut down. With reference to 1 candela per square centimeter, we are running about one quarter of that as far as discomfort glare is concerned in interior lighting.

MR. SLINEY: Fortunately, it turns out that our natural aversion response to most bright sources would tend to protect us. For instance, in testing a large number of welders it turns out that it is conventional in the welding industry to let them select their exact shade. You may prescribe a certain density, but then they will have some tolerance as to what they will permit. In almost all cases, though, when we measure the brightness of the arc and the density of the filters it turns out that they are normally selected to bring down the brightness to about 1 candela per square centimeter, which is about the brightness of sunlight on sand and is about half the brightness of sunlight on snow at noon time, which we all know is very discomforting and which, in aphakics, particularly, you can encounter cases of erythropsia, or red vision after a day of exposure to that light.

DR. LATIES: I think it is fair to point out and put some of these things in perspective, that all of our sensory systems, and really a lot of life, depends on a very delicate physical chemical balance and one of the best of possible examples is oxygen, as Dr. Noell mentioned briefly this morning.   We live in an environment which has oxygen--you can't take much more and you can't do well with much less.   It is a narrow range, but we seem to do fairly well in that narrow range for a considerable length of time.

RETINITIS PIGMENTOSA: ACCELERATED COURSE OF VISUAL LOSS SECONDARY

TO EXOGENOUS THYROID ADMINISTRATION

Jerome T. Pearlman*, J. Saxton#, and A. Van Herle#

Department of Ophthalmology, Visual Physiology Laboratory
(Retina Service), Jules Stein Eye Institute*
Department of Medicine#
UCLA School of Medicine
Los Angeles, California 90024

CASE STUDY

The following case documents the unusually rapid progression
of retinitis pigmentosa in a young woman who received, over the
course of one year, exogenous thyroid hormone for the purpose of
weight control.

A 30 year old white woman was first seen at the Jules Stein
Eye Institute in October, 1974.   She was aware at the time of her
visit that her clinical diagnosis was pigmentary degeneration of
the retina (retinitis pigmentosa) of the autosomal dominant genetic variety.   She had noticed the symptom of night blindness for
approximately ten years.   There was a positive history of retinitis
pigmentosa on the paternal side of the family with her father, two
paternal uncles, and one paternal aunt having the disease.   One
male first cousin had retinitis pigmentosa, and the male offspring
of an apparently unaffected female first cousin by the same father
was similarly affected.   The propositus has three children, aged
11, 10, and 2 years.   The 11 year old son has started to complain
of night vision difficulties, and the youngest son was born with
multiple congenital defects (Fig. 1).

The patient had a mild compound myopic astigmatism in each
eye, fully corrected to 20/20 with glasses.   External examination
was normal.   Her fundus showed the retinal pigment epithelial
changes associated with retinitis pigmentosa with some, but little
pigment in each eye.   She would be characterized as having a

223

"paucipigmentary" pattern.   Severe arteriolar attenuation and waxy
pallor of the discs were noted bilaterally.

Goldmann   visual fields showed severe peripheral constriction
compatible with the primary diagnosis.   Her electroretinogram was
non-recordable in each eye.   The first dark adaptation test,   performed on October 17, 1974, showed a 2.2 log unit elevation of
final rod threshold at the end of 45 minutes (Fig. 2, Table 1).

The patient is of particular interest because she has been
receiving exogenous thyroid medication since July or August, 1974.
This was given to her for weight control purposes by her private
internist in the community.   Initially, she began on 3 grains per
day, and the dose was gradually increased until a daily dose of 7
grains was given beginning in January, 1975.   Even at these large
doses of thyroid, the patient never appeared to overtly suffer
from symptoms of hyperthyroidism.   Clinically, however, she has
suffered from a marked increase of dental erosion and carie formation since being on this treatment (Xhonga and Van Herle, 1973).
No laboratory studies pertaining to thyroid function were performed
while the patient was on the medication.   Thus, the dental erosion
is a clue to her clinical status during that period, besides her
weight loss of 30 pounds in one year (195 lbs. to 165 lbs.), and a
pulse rate frequently recorded at 100 beats per minute.   She never
had an overt tremor, but did note some mild to moderate heat intol-
erance.   These symptoms disappeared on discontinuation of thyroid
medication.   The dental erosion, unfortunately, remains permanent.

The patient was next seen in April, 1975, when her Goldmann
fields and dark adaptation test were repeated.   These showed progressive loss of visual field, and a further elevation of the
final rod threshold by 0.2 log units (Fig. 3, Table 1).   The
patient was still being maintained on 7 grains of thyroid per day.

Her third visit was in May, 1975, at which time she showed
yet further deterioration of her visual fields, and an additional
elevation of her rod threshold by 0.6 log units (Fig. 4, Table 1).
Thus, with respect to her dark adaptation function, there was a
0.8 log unit change in rod threshold between October, 1974, and
May, 1975. At this point, the patient was instructed, through her
internist, to discontinue thyroid medication.

Her fourth visit, in September, 1975, revealed even further
progression of visual field loss, but some slight improvement of
her dark adaptation function (Fig. 5, Table 1). By comparison
with her previous dark adaptation test, which showed a 3.0 log
unit elevation of rod threshold, the test showed only a 2.6 log
unit elevation, or an improvement of 0.4 log units (2 S.D. = ± 0.6
log units for our laboratory). Subjectively, the patient felt her
night vision had improved.   The continued deterioration of the

visual field could be accounted for on the basis of a continued
influence of the thyroid medication, even one and one half to two
months after its cessation.

At the time of her most recent visit, in November, 1975, there
was a slight improvement in her visual fields and in her dark adapted threshold (Fig. 6, Table 1). The latter test showed a 2.3 log
unit elevation of final rod threshold.

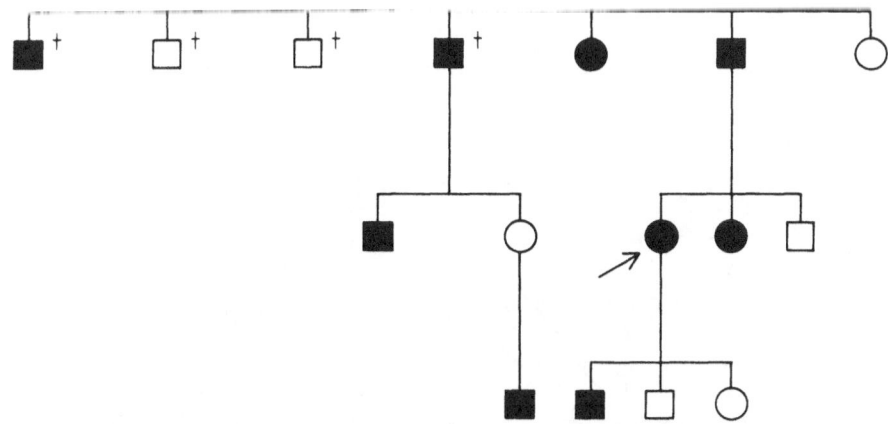

FIGURE 1. Pedigree showing autosomal dominant hereditary transmission. Black squares represent affected males; black circles,
affected females. The arrow designates the propositus.

Further follow-up testing will continue for one year, at two
to three month intervals, and thereafter at six month intervals.

Thyroid studies performed in November, 1975, consisted of a 24
hour I-131 uptake (5%), considered in the low range of normal; a
normal thyroid scan; a T-3 resin uptake of 38.3% (normal range =
35-45%); and T-4 (by column) of 5.0 micrograms/100 ml (normal = 2.9
to 6.4). Sedimentation rate, alkaline phosphatase, creatinine,
uric acid, urea nitrogen, total cholesterol, glucose, SGO trans-
aminase, hematocrit, and routine blood studies were all normal.

COMMENT AND DISCUSSION

Pigmentary retinal degeneration, more commonly known as
"retinitis pigmentosa," refers to a group of variously inherited
disorders characterized by night blindness, severe constriction of
the peripheral visual fields, marked attenuation of the retinal
arterioles, and waxy pallor of the optic disc. Characteristically,
the disease is slowly progressive over a course of many years, and
may take decades before resulting in total blindness. Visual
fields, though impaired, may remain stable for long periods of
time. Then, there may be other times when there is more rapid progression of visual field deterioration. The factors responsible
for the more rapid progression of the disease are not known, but
pregnancy in women affected with retinitis pigmentosa appears to

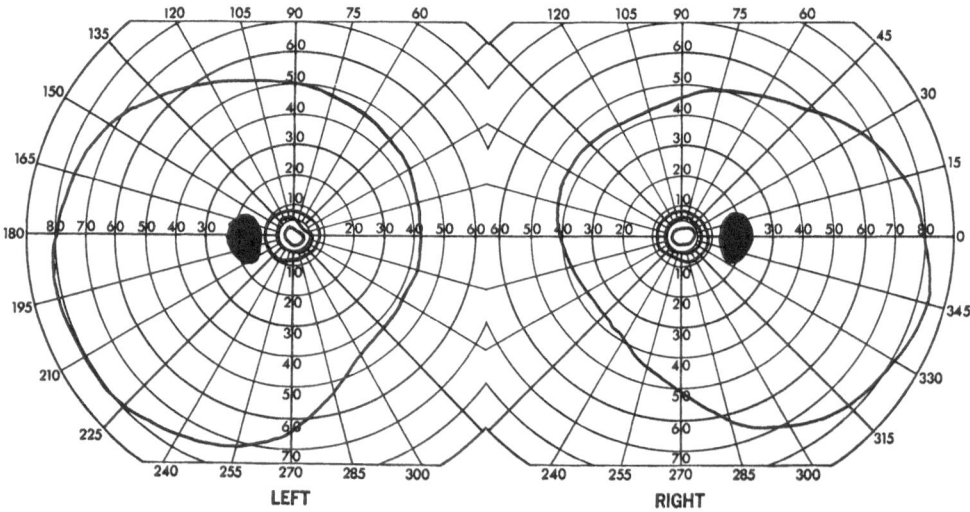

FIGURE 2. Goldmann fields, October, 1974. The first test performed.

have a deleterious effect in a number of cases (Pearlman and Saxton, 1975). The influence of ambient light, particularly bright
or glare light, could also, on theoretical grounds, result in the
more rapid progression of the disease (Dowling and Sidman, 1962).
Doubtless, there are other factors as yet incompletely understood
that may have an equally adverse influence. In a culture such as
ours, where an enormous variety of drugs and medications are prescribed and taken for a multiplicity of reasons, attention must be
given to the possible deleterious effect that such agents might
exert on the progressive course of a disease unrelated to the reason for giving medication.

Diagnostic tests performed to establish the presence of
retinitis pigmentosa include fundus examination, fluorescein angiography, electrooculography, electroretinography, visual field
testing, and dark adaptometry. Of these, the last three, perhaps,
are the most widely used of the special diagnostic tests apart from
the usual information derived from fundus examination by ophthal-
moscopy. Characteristically, the electroretinogram, which is a
measurement of the action potential of the retina in response to
brief flashes of light, is highly impaired or non-recordable in the
early stages of the disease. Visual fields show a severe restriction of peripheral vision, resulting in tubular or "tunnel" vision
with the preservation of central visual acuity. Dark adaptometry,
or the measurement of the absolute threshold to dim light stimulation following a period of glare light stimulation, is of great
value in following the progression of the disease by quantitating

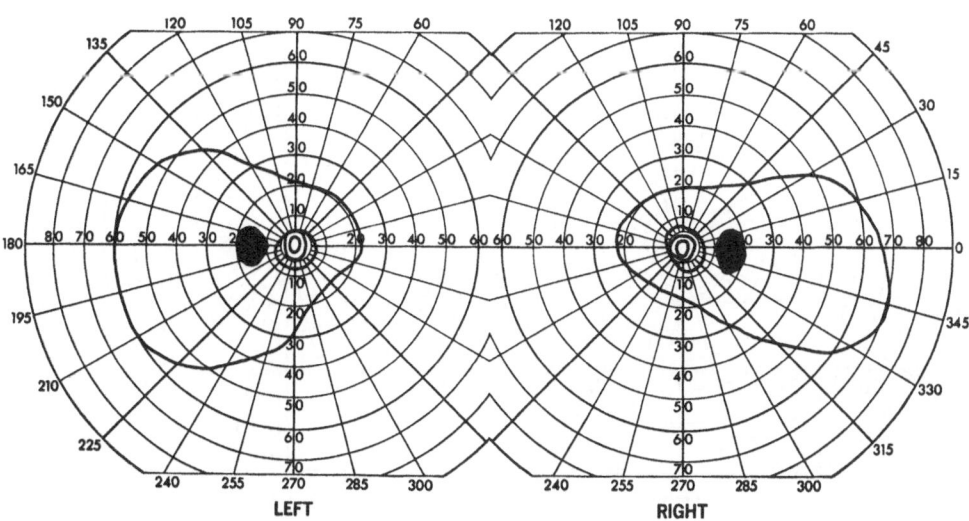

FIGURE 3. Goldmann fields, April, 1975. The second test showing
    further constriction of smaller isopters.

the loss of rod function. Since the electroretinogram is severely
impaired early in the course of the disease, it cannot be used
effectively as a test to monitor progression.   This leaves visual
field examination and dark adaptometry as the mainstay of follow-
up examinations.

Such a rapid progression of clinical symptoms is unusual for
a person in whom the mode of hereditary transmission is autosomal
dominant.   Usually, this form of retinitis pigmentosa, occurring
later in life, is milder and more slowly progressive (Allan, 1937;
Franceschetti *et al.*, 1974). The field changes and the dark adaptometry changes noted here are very marked.

This case is one that has been anticipated for a long while,
on theoretical grounds. It has been suspected that thyroid hormone
may have an adverse influence on patients with retinitis pigmentosa, in the same fashion that birth control pills and pregnancy
may cause the disease to progress at an accelerated rate (Pearlman
and Saxton, 1975).

So far, in the several hundred patients that have been examined with retinitis pigmentosa over the past six or seven years,
no individual has appeared with a history of having taken significant amounts of thyroid hormone for medical purposes.

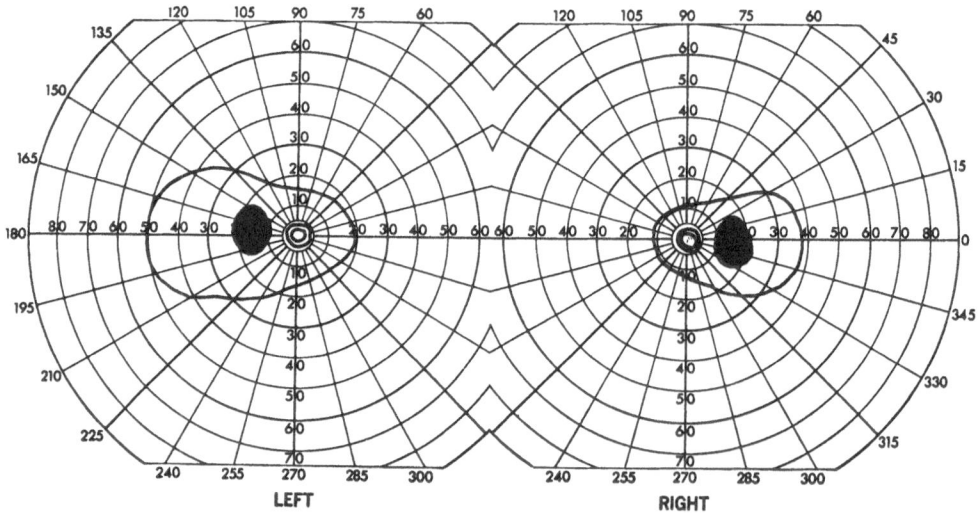

FIGURE 4. Goldmann fields, May, 1975. The third test showing even
   more marked field loss.

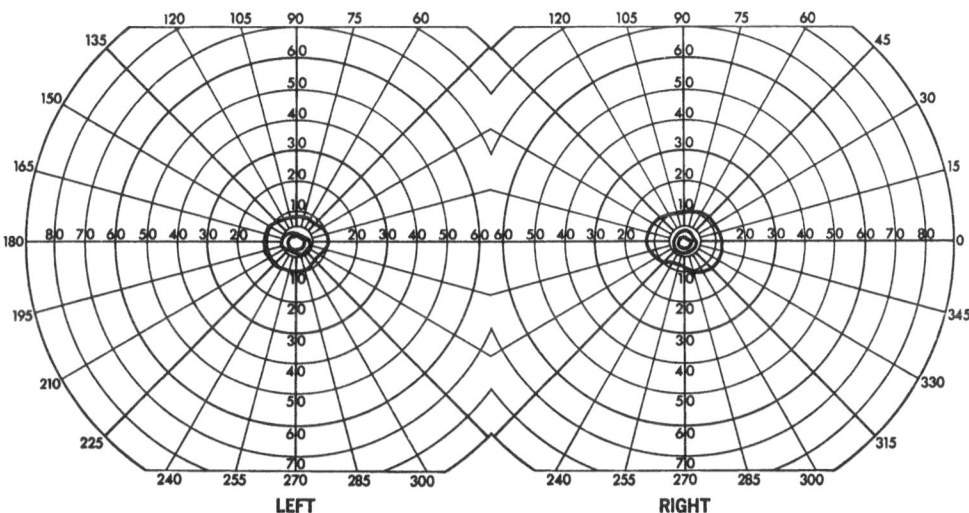

FIGURE 5. Goldmann fields, September, 1975. The first test after
discontinuing thyroid medication. Field loss continues as a
residual effect of the drug. There is a slight improvement of
the corresponding final rod threshold

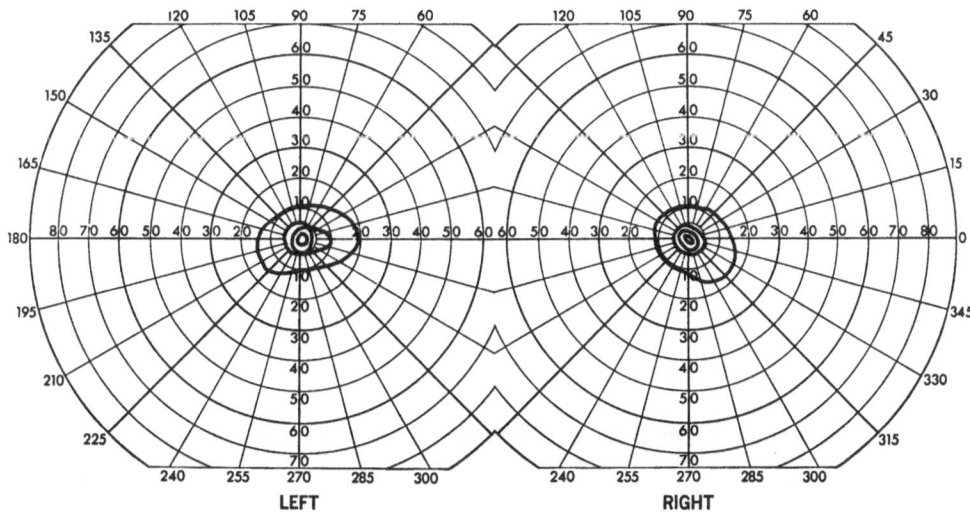

FIGURE 6. Goldmann fields, November, 1975. The second test
after discontinuing thyroid medication, showing some further
improvement, together with lowered rod threshold by dark adaptation.

TABLE I

ELEVATION OF FINAL ROD THRESHOLD
WITH DARK ADAPTATION AT DIFFERENT EXAMINATION TIMES

Date	Elevation of final (40-45 min) rod threshold on dark adaptation (log units)
October 1974	2.2
April 1975	2.4
May 1975	3.0
(Thyroid medication stopped mid-May 1975)	
September 1975	2.6
October 1975	2.3

The mode of action of thyroid upon the retina is not known, but the hormone characteristically has the ability of accelerating metabolic activity throughout the entire body. It seems feasible that such an influence may have an adverse effect on a rod system which is already impaired, either by its inability to dispose of cast-off outer segment tips from the rods (Young and Bok, 1969; Herron *et al.*, 1969; Bok and Hall, 1971), or by problems of outer segment renewal as has been suggested by Young (1977), or by the deleterious effect of elevated body temperature (Noell *et al.*, 1966; Wolbarsht *et al.*, 1977).

Animal studies are currently under way to determine whether thyroid administration or deprivation can alter the time course of genetically determined retinal dystrophy.

Finally, if one had a patient with retinitis pigmentosa who began to show an unusually rapid acceleration of peripheral field loss and night vision difficulty, it would be an excellent idea to check the patient's thyroid status to see whether there was a concurrent hyperthyroidism. Grave's disease is treatable, and the implications for vision in a patient with retinitis pigmentosa might be very significant.

SUMMARY

A 30 year old white female with known retinitis pigmentosa of autosomal dominant transmission was placed on thyroid medication for weight control purposes for nearly one year. The unusually rapid progression of visual field changes and the increased severity of night vision problems are documented by serial functional studies.

ACKNOWLEDGEMENTS

The authors gratefully acknowledge the technical assistance of Nola J. Allston, Robert Petrus, and Gwynne Gloege, Edward Allen, and Jay Sands. This study was supported by NIH grant EY 00331 from the National Eye Institute (Bethesda, Maryland), and from the private contributions of the Sklar and Phillips Families (Shreveport, Louisiana).

REFERENCES

Allan, W. (1937) Eugenic significance of retinitis pigmentosa. *Arch. Ophthal.* 18:938-947.

Bok, D., and Hall, M. O. (1971) The role of the pigment epithelium in the etiology of inherited retinal dystrophy in the rat. *J. Cell Biol.* 49:664-682.

Dowling, J. E., and Sidman, R. L. (1962) Inherited retinal dystrophy in the rat. *J. Cell Biol.* 14:73-109.

Franceschetti, A., Francois, J., and Babel, J. (1974) "Chorioretinal Heredo-Degenerations" p. 204, Charles C Thomas, Springfield, Ill.

Herron, W. L., Jr., Riegel, B. W., Meyers, O. E., and Rubin, M. L. (1969) Retinal dystrophy in the rat--a pigment epithelial disease. *Invest. Ophthal.* 8:595-604.

Wolbarsht, M. L., Landers, M. B., III, Wadsworth, J. A. C., and Anderson, W. B., Jr. (1977) Retinitis pigmentosa: clinical management based on current concepts, in "Retinitis Pigmentosa: Clinical Implications of Current Research" (M. B. Landers, M. L. Wolbarsht, J. E. Dowling, and A. M. Laties, eds.) Plenum Press, New York.

Noell, W. K., Walker, V. S., Kang, B. S., and Berman, S. (1966) Retinal damage by light in rats. *Invest. Ophthal.* 5:450-473.

Pearlman, J., and Saxton, J. (1975) Retinitis pigmentosa and birth
    control pills. *J. Amer. Med. Assoc.* 231(8):810.

Young, R. W. (1977) Visual cell renewal systems and the problem
    of retinitis pigmentosa, in "Retinitis Pigmentosa: Clinical
    Implications of Current Research" (M. B. Landers, M. L. Wol-
    barsht, J. E. Dowling, and A. E. Laties, eds.) pp. 93-113,
    Plenum Press, New York.

Young, R. W., and Bok, D. (1969) Participation of the retinal pig-
    ment epithelium in the rod outer segment renewal process. *J.
    Cell. Biol.* 42:392-403.

Xhonga, F. A., and Van Herle, A. (1973) The influence of hyperthy-
    roidism on dental erosions. *Oral Surg., Oral Med., Oral Path.*
    36:349-357

PROTECTION AGAINST PHOTIC DAMAGE IN RETINITIS PIGMENTOSA

Werner Adrian*, Ronald W. Everson, and Ingeborg Schmidt

Lighttechnical Institute*
University of Karlsruhe
Karlsruhe, West Germany

School of Optometry
Indiana University
Bloomington, Indiana 47401

INTRODUCTION

The research described here was initiated after a student asked us, on behalf of his brother who suffers from retinitis pigmentosa (RP), whether or not there was a cure for the disease. Inquiries and literature studies revealed that sporadic successes have been reported with drugs (vitamins, vasodilators, RNA) or with operations (sympathectomy), but that none has given a lasting effect. However, experiments on rats (which demonstrated that protection from light, if started early, did decelerate degeneration of their retinas) suggested a method to explore for its possible benefit to humans.

EVIDENCE FOR PHOTIC RETINAL DAMAGE

Experiments on rats with hereditary retinal dystrophy, which is very similar to human RP, have shown that exposure to light accelerates the retinal degeneration and that keeping the animals in total darkness delays, but does not arrest, the degeneration. The degree of retinal damage was ascertained by changes in the electroretinogram (ERG), by the rhodopsin content of the retina, and by histopathological examination (Dowling and Sidman, 1962; Dowling, 1964; Noell, 1965).

In addition, several authors (Gorn and Kuwabara, 1967; Kuwabara and Gorn, 1968; Noell, 1965; Noell *et al*., 1966, 1971; Noell and Albrecht, 1971) have investigated the effect of illumination

233

on the retinas of normal rats. Because the normal rat retina is
very sensitive to light, the experimenters produced damage which
depended on intensity, spectral composition (the results corresponding to the bleaching effect of colored lights on visual purple),
duration of illumination, and duration of recovery periods. A
sudden change from darkness to continuous bright light was especially damaging. The higher the body temperature above normal, the
shorter the time required for the light of given intensity to produce an effect. However, normal rat retinas were more resistant to
damage by light than were degenerating retinas.

The retina of the rat is almost a pure rod retina. In 1973,
Berson reported on experiments on ground squirrels--animals which
have pure cone retinas. Ground squirrels which were fed a normal
diet did not demonstrate any effects, but vitamin A deficient animals showed some retinal damage due to illumination. Cone retinas
appeared to be far more resistant to photic injury than rod retinas.

Experiments on photic damage to retinas containing rods and
cones in animals with hereditary retinal dystrophy have not been
performed to our knowledge.

It is obviously difficult to say how much of the knowledge
obtained from the experiments on animals, especially from those on
rats which have a rod retina that is very sensitive to light, can
be extrapolated to humans. If it were possible to demonstrate
statistically that human RP progresses more quickly in sunny southern countries than in northern ones, this would be evidence for an
effect of photic damage. But up to now such comparative studies
have not been possible because of the uneven distribution of the
disease and the fact that there are several forms of RP with
different rates of progress. There is, however, some clinical
evidence which supports the assumption that illumination may accelerate degeneration of the retina in human RP. In many cases, the
upper visual field, corresponding to the lower retina, disappears
earlier than the lower field (sometimes it is more the upper nasal
field, sometimes the upper temporal field). In fact, the lower
field can still be normal. Also, typical textbook pictures frequently show that the lower half of the fundus in RP exhibits more
pathological pigmentation than the upper. One may speculate at
least that these effects occur because the lower retina gets more
intense illumination than the upper, e.g., from the sky or overhead
lights. In addition, vision may be retained longer in the far
periphery of the retina because its illumination is lower than that
of more central regions (Leber, 1916).

There is also some clinical evidence demonstrating that in
human RP the rods are affected earlier and to a greater extent
than the cones. A functional deficiency of the rods occurs far

before any noticeable malfunction of the cones, namely, disturbed night vision as a first subjective symptom of the disease. This is clearly demonstrated by the more pronounced elevation of the rod than the cone threshold in the dark adaptation curve. Moreover, the ring scotoma forms where the rod population in the retina is most dense, while good central vision by cones is usually retained for some time.

However, that the cones, too, are already affected in the beginning stages of all types of inherited RP has been shown by electrophysiological tests (Berson, 1973). Light microscopic (Cogan, 1950) and electron microscopic (Mizuno and Nishida, 1967) examinations of human retinas in an advanced stage of the disease have demonstrated that the cones are the last to disappear.

PROTECTION FROM PHOTIC RETINAL DAMAGE

The observations reported allow one to hypothesize that light may be a factor in the progress of human RP and that the human rods will degenerate more rapidly than the cones. Therefore, one could try to protect the retinas of RP patients from bright general illumination in the hope of decelerating the course of the disease. It would seem prudent to protect the rods to a greater extent than the cones.

The protection could take the form of dark ophthalmic filters which would meet several theoretical criteria.

Criteria for a Protective Device

1. The total light transmittance should be low, as low as is compatible with the wearer's ordinary visual tasks, in order to protect the retina from bright light. The lenses should not be so dark as to handicap the patient, lest they then not be worn. As long as no specific data are available, it appears reasonable to specify a total luminous transmittance of approximately 10% for an ophthalmic filter used outdoors and of a somewhat higher level for use indoors. RP patients with appreciably constricted visual fields probably would require more light transmission than these levels, but the point is moot, because it is questionable whether protection from light would be of benefit in already advanced degenerations.

2. The spectral characteristics of the ophthalmic filter should be such as to protect the rods to a greater extent than the cones. This can be achieved by selecting a material of such spectral transmission that only a small fraction of the light entering the eye is absorbed by the rods.

Adrian (Adrian and Schmidt, 1975a) quantified this criterion by computing a cone/rod ratio, R, of the portions of the incident light which serve as stimuli for the cones and rods, respectively. If one assumes a light source with an equal energy spectrum and a standard observer, the stimulus value (illuminance) for the cone pigments of the unfiltered incident light is proportional to the area, A, under the CIE photopic luminosity curve. The stimulus value of the light transmitted by the ophthalmic filter is proportional to a portion, a, of that area. The relative stimulus value of the transmitted light for the cone pigments is then the ratio, a/A. In the same manner, the relative stimulus value of the transmitted light for the rod pigment is the ratio, b/B, where b is that portion of the total area, B, under the CIE scotopic luminosity curve, which is proportional to the quantity of transmitted light. Finally, the ratio, R, of the relative stimulation of cones to rods is equal to a/A ÷ b/B, or a/b · B/A. For any other than an equal energy source, the spectral radiant flux density (emittance) of the source must be incorporated.

The ratio, R, is computed from the following equation, which corresponds to R = a/b · B/A:

$$R = \frac{\int Le\lambda \cdot T(\lambda) \cdot V(\lambda) d\lambda}{\int Le\lambda \cdot T(\lambda) \; V'(\lambda) d\lambda} \cdot \frac{\int Le\lambda \cdot V'(\lambda) d\lambda}{\int Le\lambda \cdot V(\lambda) d\lambda}$$

where $V(\lambda)$ = CIE photopic luminosity factor; $V'(\lambda)$ = CIE scotopic luminosity factor; $T(\lambda)$ = spectral transmittance of the filter; $Le\lambda$ = spectral radiant flux density of the incident light.

A neutral gray filter transilluminated by light from an equal energy spectrum has a ratio, R, of 1.0. A blue filter, which preferentially transmits short visible wavelengths, has a ratio less than 1.0. The wavelengths transmitted are those to which the rods are more sensitive than the cones. Filters which transmit mainly long visible wavelengths have ratios above 1.0. The cones are more sensitive than the rods to these wavelengths.

For the purpose of relative protection of the rods, the cone/rod ratio, R, should be as high as is compatible with useful vision.

Red filters which transmit only the longest visible wavelengths would have very high cone/rod ratios. However, red glasses usually are not acceptable for full time wear. The patient may not become accustomed to the monotony of the red surround and may refuse to wear the filters even though the redness would be diminished somewhat by the color constancy phenomenon. Moreover, the wavelengths transmitted by a filter should allow at least a small degree of color discrimination, especially differentiation of red and green for reasons of traffic safety, but this would not be possible with a red filter. This leads to the next criterion for the protective device.

3. The reduction of color discrimination through the ophthalmic filter should be as minimal as possible and at the very least the filter should permit correct identification of traffic signals. This is important for both pedestrian and motorist.

4. In the visible regions, absorption of ultraviolet and infrared would seem to be advantageous.

5. The filter material must meet certain standards. It is desirable that prescription power can be incorporated if required. Alternatively, the glasses could be fitover goggles to be worn in combination with corrective lenses. The optical quality of the filter should be high so that long wear does not cause asthenopic symptoms. Also, the material should not deteriorate with time or exposure.

6. The spectacle frame should have large side shields which are opaque or of low light transmittance, and also have a rim across the top, to afford protection against obliquely-incident light. If frames are not supplied with such devices, simple modifications can sometimes be made to them. Spectacle frames are available for industrial use which have dark colors and side shields. If fitover goggles are necessary, they should fit well and comfortably over the corrective glasses. This problem, of course, does not exist for individuals who wear their corrections in the form of contact lenses.

7. From the viewpoint of the patient, the glasses should be cosmetically acceptable.

The Adrian Filter

By adhering to these criteria as far as possible, one of the authors, Adrian, assembled a combination of Kodak Wratten filters which gave a spectral transmittance curve very similar to curve A in Fig. 1, which is actually that of a later, glass design (Adrian and Schmidt, 1975b). No light is transmitted by the filter below wavelength 540 nm in order to protect the rod pigment. Long wavelengths which are not capable of bleaching rhodopsin significantly are fully transmitted. A band of transmission about 100 nm wide in the green-yellow region is added to enlarge the array of colors perceptible through the filter. This is essential for discrimination of red and green. The transmittance in the green-yellow band is kept low to minimize the stimulation of the rods by these visible wavelengths and to keep the total luminous transmittance of the filter low.

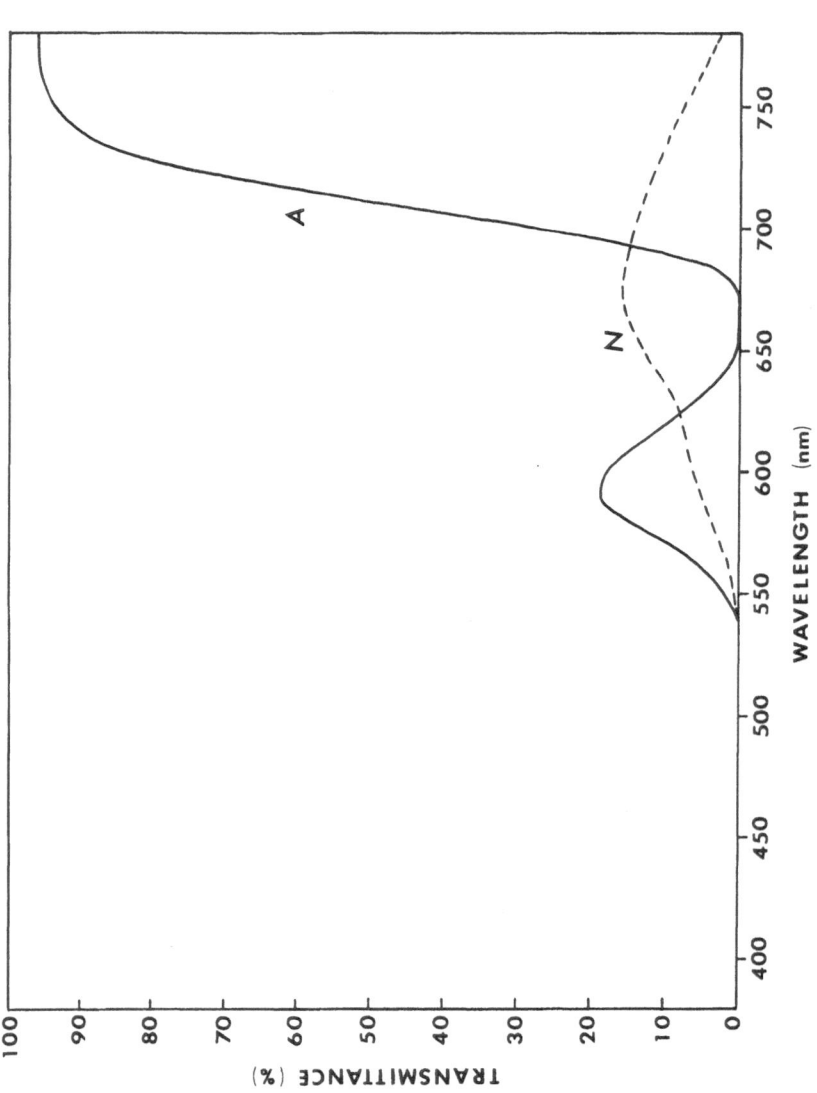

FIGURE 1. Spectral transmission curves of A, the Adrian Lens (second design), and N, the NoIR Amber 7% Filter.

The original design enclosed three Kodak Wratten gelatin filters between glass. Later, the combination was replaced by commercially prepared lenses having an absorptive layer between two pieces of glass with antireflective coatings on the outer surfaces. The latter lenses are manufactured by the Carl Zeiss Company in Aalen, West Germany. They have a brownish appearance, a total light transmittance of 6.9% for daylight, and a cone/rod ratio, R, of 7.6.

The retinitis pigmentosa patient mentioned in the Introduction, a male 22 years of age, was fitted with the combination design and later the glass design of the protective filter. The ametropic correction was incorporated in the glasses. The patient's visual acuity with correction was 20/20 O.D., 20/60 O.S. His left eye has had reduced visual acuity since birth. Figure 2 demonstrates the visual field of the right eye taken on different dates by one of the authors. A comparison of the field taken in November, 1969 with that taken in June, 1970 shows that the disease must have been active during this period. This was confirmed by his ophthalmologist. In June, 1970 the patient began wearing the protective filters. He was instructed to wear them not only outdoors, but also in brightly lit rooms. When measured again in January, 1972, the visual field was enlarged, almost up to the extent established in November, 1969. However, it is not possible to ascribe this to the filters because the observed improvement may have been one of the spontaneous regressions known to occur in this disease. We also do not know whether or not there is a possibility of seasonal fluctuations of the visual fields in RP depending upon the outdoor illumination, with an enlarged field in winter and a smaller one in summer.

Evaluation of Other Filters

Because of complications in the procedure for obtaining material from overseas, a search was begun for ophthalmic filters available in this country which could serve as temporary or even permanent substitutes for the Adrian filter. Such filters would have a brownish to reddish appearance.

Samples of brown ophthalmic filters were gathered from a number of sources, including standard ophthalmic suppliers as well as from nonprescription sunglass displays. Some filters were promptly set aside after initial tests revealed that they did not approach the special requirements already described.

A common feature of nonprescription sunglasses is their high luminous transmittance which makes even those which are brown and reddish-brown unsuitable for protection of RP patients.

The Photobrown lenses by Corning were initially considered for their ability to adjust transmittance to the ambient light level. However, for purposes of protection in RP, their luminous transmittance is too high for use outdoors and they do not darken enough for such use indoors. In sunlight, a Photobrown lens of 2 mm thickness has approximately 45% transmittance. The lenses also transmit an appreciable quantity of light of short wavelengths.

The following ophthalmic filters were given close inspection. Plastic lenses: NoIR Model 101 Amber 14%, NoIR Model 107 Amber 7%, both available only in fitover goggle form from the Recreational Innovations Company, Medical Products Division, and an experimental clear plastic lens which was dipped in both brown and gray dyes at our request by a prescription optical laboratory. Glass lenses: Meyer-Tan C from the Meyer Optical Company, Nutra-Tone Brown No. 4 Coating from Pacific Universal Products Corporation, and Bausch and Lomb's Didymium G-20 lens which was given a brown coating.

Measurements as follows were made on these filters:

1. Luminous transmittance under a Macbeth daylight illuminant by means of a Knick Photoelectric Meter. Transmittances under incandescent and fluorescent illuminants were also obtained and were within 3% of those for daylight.

2. Spectral transmission curve for the visible spectrum by means of a Bausch and Lomb Spectrophotometer. From the curves the filters' R ratios were calculated for an equal energy spectrum. The calculations were made in intervals of 1 nm.

3. Visual performance through the filters; namely, visual acuity and color naming experiments were performed.

Detailed results including figures of spectral transmission curves have been reported (Everson and Schmidt, 1976). The results show that of the tested filters only the NoIR lenses have characteristics which resemble the Adrian lens.

The NoIR Amber 14% has a luminous transmittance for daylight of 10.9% and a cone/rod ratio, R, of 4.0. The NoIR Amber 7% has a luminous transmittance of 5.6% for daylight and a cone/rod ratio, R, of 12.1. The latter has the highest R ratio of all filters evaluated. The spectral transmission curve of the NoIR Amber 7% filter is shown in Fig. 1. That these filters absorb infrared may be an additional advantage.

The NoIR lenses are supplied as integral, nonremovable parts of large frames which can be worn over corrective glasses. Their appearance is modern and acceptable. The optical qualities of the surfaces of the NoIR lenses, judged from images reflected from

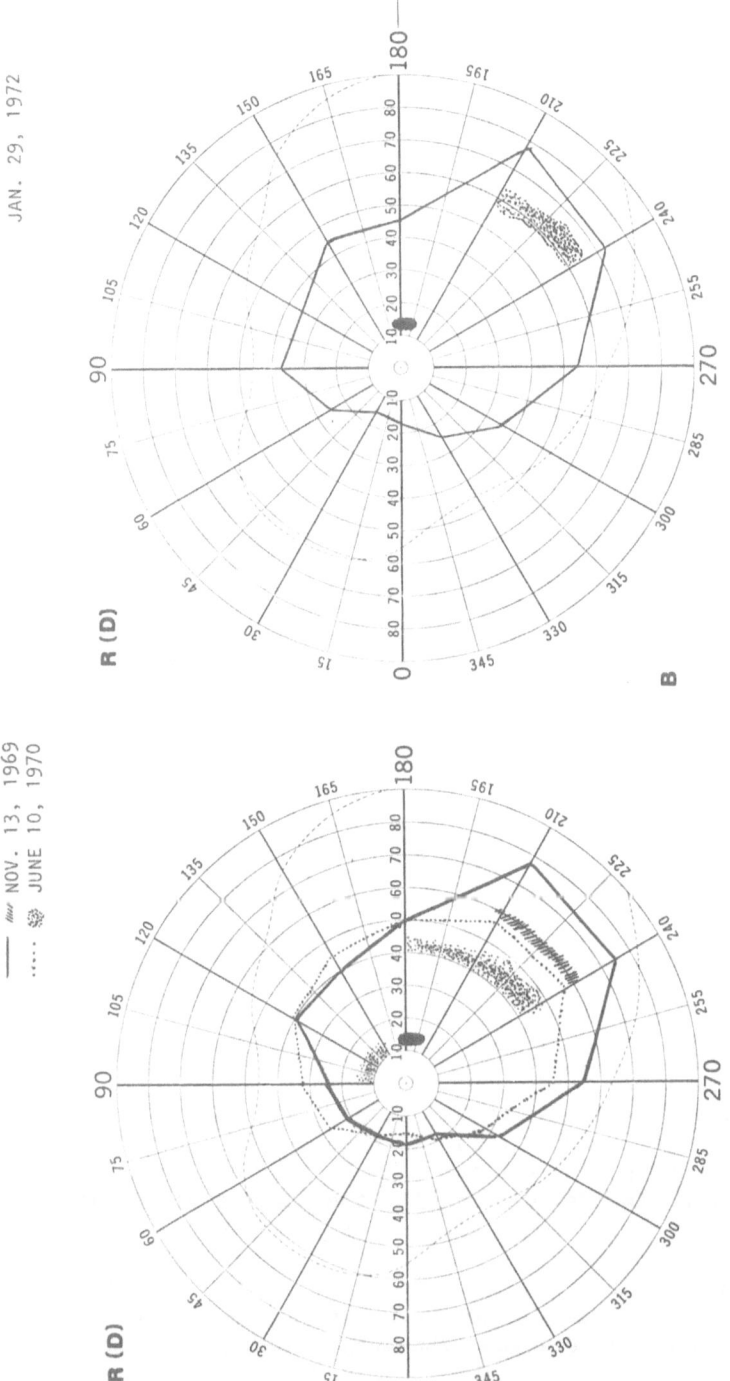

FIGURE 2. Visual fields of the right eye of RP patient, measured with a Zeiss-Maggiore pro-
jection perimeter. Object 6/333 mm, white, intensity 1.0. Chart A: Before wearing
the protective ophthalmic filter; fields measured in November 1969 (solid lines) and
June 1970 (dotted lines). Chart B: Field measured in January 1972, after having worn
the protective filters for one and one-half years.

them, are far superior to those of some inexpensive, nonprescription plastic sunglasses. Another advantage of the NoIR glasses is that they have wide temples which double as side shields, the temples and frames being of the same transparent brown plastic as the lenses, thus permitting utilization and protection of the peripheral fields. To some extent, the upper rim of the frames also protects from light incident from above. The NoIR Amber 7% filters are in fact recommended by the manufacturer (Recreational Innovations Company, 1974) for use with albinos and RP patients. The disadvantage of the NoIR glasses and of plastic lenses in general is that they scratch more easily than do glass lenses. There is also the familiar problem of wearing the glasses over corrective lenses, and the frames are not especially durable.

Comparison of the Adrian and the NoIR Amber 7% Filters

When looking alternately through the two filters, one can observe that details are more sharply defined and contrasts are more distinct through the Adrian glass lens than through the NoIR Amber 7% lens. On longer wear the Adrian lens is the more comfortable of the two. The environment appears slightly discolored through both. Through both lenses, but somewhat more effectively through the Adrian lens, the phenomenon of color constancy restores a more natural appearance in a short time.

In a field test, traffic signals of red, yellow, and green could be distinguished from a distance of 300 feet (91 m) through both filters.

These preliminary observations prompted further investigation of the effect of the two filters on visual performance. They were studied in comparison with a Kodak Wratten Neutral Density 1.1 filter, the transmittance of which (7.9%) was close to that of the two filters.

Visual acuity with the filters. A Clason Acuity Meter was used to measure the visual acuity of four subjects, three males and one female, ages 23-24, while they viewed the projected target from a distance of 20 feet (6 m) through the filters. The target was a grating having fine vertical lines. The room was semi-dark. Before the measurements were made, the subject was allowed five minutes of adaptation through each filter.

Although the difference was very small, visual acuity for each of the four subjects was better with the Adrian filter than with the NoIR 7%. Both filters gave the subjects slightly better visual acuity than did the neutral density filter.

TABLE I

AVERAGE SCORES ON THE SAM COLOR THRESHOLD TESTER

Signal Color	Scores for Each Type of Lens		
	Adrian	NoIR 7%	N.D. 1.1
Red	6.16	6.50	5.16
Green	4.50	5.50	5.66
Yellow	7.00	6.17	7.00
Orange	7.00	5.33	6.66
Blue	0.00	0.83	1.83
White	3.66	2.33	6.33

Color naming with the filters. The ability to discriminate colors of lights was studied on a signal lantern, the SAM Color Threshold Tester, designed by L. L. Sloan for Air Force pilot selection (Sloan, 1944). The instructions for its use were closely followed. The data obtained at the lowest intensity were omitted because the low transmittances of the filters dimmed the signal lights so much that they were at or below the threshold of seeing. When a color was named correctly at all seven remaining intensities, the subject's score was 7.0. Six males, all normal trichromats, ages 23 to 27 years, were subjects. The average scores on six colors are given in Table I. The order of wearing the three filters was randomized among the subjects.

The scores demonstrate that the NoIR Amber 7% and the Adrian lens were approximately equal in permitting recognition of red, the NoIR filter being only slightly superior. Both were superior to the neutral density filter in this respect, which is understandable because they transmit more red light than the latter. In the recognition of green, the Adrian lens was inferior because it made green appear whitish. Yellow and orange were recognized without mistake through the Adrian lens, whereas through the NoIR Amber 7%, orange was occasionally called red. The white signal light was mistakenly called orange frequently through both filters. Blue was barely perceived, even through the neutral density filter. None of the filters caused a confusion of red with green. The misinterpretations mentioned cannot be regarded as dangerous and probably would be readily compensated by learning.

Compared to the NoIR Amber 7% filter, the Adrian lens has the advantage that it can be ground to prescription and mounted in a choice of spectacle frames. The NoIR lens has the advantage that it is readily available. Both permit discrimination of traffic signals.

Other Recommendations for Protection

In addition to using ophthalmic filters, individuals can obtain protection from overhead light outdoors by wearing a hat with a large brim. For indoor use, conventional brown, amber, or orange sunglasses with moderate luminous transmittances may be sufficient because indoor illumination is at a much lower level than outdoor illumination. Also, it has lower color temperature than skylight, containing a smaller proportion of short wavelength light. Moreover, there are other means of modifying indoor illumination, e.g., brown-tinted lamp shades, reduced-wattage bulbs, yellow bulbs, etc.

DISCUSSION OF RELATED PROBLEMS AND SUGGESTIONS

It is an open question whether or not it is better to protect both eyes from light and thus try to decelerate the degeneration of both eyes simultaneously, or, as Berson (1971) has suggested, to cover one eye light-tight with a flush-fitting opaque scleral contact lens in an effort to keep this eye in reserve while the other eye exposed normally to light degenerates in the usual course of the disease.

Monocular vision produced by occluding one eye has several disadvantages. When using only one eye the patient may be unable to drive a car because he cannot fill in his defective visual field with the field of the other eye. Binocular fields would reduce this difficulty as long as the two fields were not exactly superimposed. Moreover, the monocular patient would not have stereoscopic vision, although he would learn to compensate for this deficiency. In addition, it is not known how fast an eye kept in darkness for years will degenerate upon re-exposure to light. The use of ophthalmic filters binocularly would create an exposure to "cyclic light," which may be beneficial. With the filters, the light phase would be at low illumination which, however, is not precisely controllable because of variable illumination of the environment. There is also a question about which method would cause greater hardship to the patient--to live with the absence of one visual impression in normal illumination or to live binocularly under reduced illumination. The monocular method probably would be carried out more strictly by the patient. It is easier to remove and replace spectacles than to insert a scleral contact lens; thus, the patient may be more negligent with the spectacles.

We do not know yet how effective light protection will be for humans. If the animal studies can be carried over to humans, they suggest that patients with primary RP should avoid bright illumination and particularly sudden changes from dark to bright. Clinicians should omit the bright adaptation period at the beginning of a dark adaptation examination. A light adaptation becomes unnecessary when applying a method suggested by Sloan (1939) as being particularly suited for testing RP patients, namely, testing the light threshold at different retinal regions in the fully dark-adapted eye. In a teaching clinic, one should probably not let a large group of observers perform successive ophthalmoscopic examinations on RP patients. Also, dilatation of the pupils should be carefully considered with regard to the consequent retinal illumination.

SUMMARY AND CONCLUSIONS

Experiments on photic damage to the retinas of rats with hereditary retinal dystrophy and some tentative clinical evidence on human patients suggest that, in human retinitis pigmentosa, one could try to protect the retina and especially the rods from bright light in an attempt to delay the retinal degeneration and to prolong the period of useful vision. Several theoretical criteria have been proposed for protection of RP patients from possible photic retinal damage. Observing these criteria, Adrian developed a brownish ophthalmic filter which absorbs the short wavelengths preferentially, thus protecting the rods primarily. Whether or not use of these filters will be efficacious has yet to be determined and will require careful experimentation and the accumulation of clinical experience. Several brown ophthalmic filters also have been tested against the criteria for a protective device. The NoIR Amber 7% plastic glasses satisfy these criteria quite well and thus can be considered as a substitute for the Adrian lens. The characteristics of the two types of filters are compared. Experience with different methods of protection may show whether it is better to attempt to delay degeneration of both retinas simultaneously by decreasing their illuminations with filters or to exclude light completely from one eye in an attempt to preserve it while the other eye degenerates in the usual course of the disease. In any event, given the present state of knowledge, it seems to be appropriate, especially in the early stages of the disease, to suggest that RP patients protect their retinas from excessive light.

REFERENCES

Adrian, W., and Schmidt, I. (1975a) Photische Schädigung der Reti-
    na bei primärer Pigmentdegeneration und mögliche Abhilfen.
    Klinische Monatsblätter für Augenheilkunde 164:744.

Adrian, W., and Schmidt, I. (1975b) Photic damage in retinitis pig-
    mentosa and a suggestion for a protective device. *J. Amer.
    Optom. Assoc.* 46:380.

Berson, E. L. (1971) Light deprivation for early retinitis pigmen-
    tosa: an hypothesis. *Arch. Ophthal.* 85:521.

Berson, E. L. (1973) Experimental and therapeutic aspects of pho-
    tic damage to the retina. *Invest. Ophthal.* 12:35.

Cogan, D. G. (1950)   Pathology.   *Trans. Amer. Acad. Ophthal. Oto-
    laryngol.* 54:629.

Dowling, J. E.   (1964)   Nutritional   and   inherited   blindness in
    the rat. *Exp. Eye Res.* 3:348.

Dowling, J. E., and Sidman, R. L. (1962)   Inherited retinal dys-
    trophy in rats. *J. Cell. Biol.* 14:73.

Everson, R. W., and Schmidt, I. (1976)   Protective spectacles for
    retinitis pigmentosa patients. *J. Amer. Optom. Assoc.* 47:738.

Gorn, R. A., and Kuwabara, T. (1967)   Retinal damage by visible
    light. *Arch. Ophthal.* 77:155.

Kuwabara, T., and Gorn, R. A. (1968)   Retinal damage by visible
    light. *Arch. Ophthal.* 79:69.

Leber, T. (1916)   Die Pigmentdegeneration der Netzhaut und mit ihr
    verwandte Erkrankungen, in "Graefe-Saemisch-Hess Handbuch d.
    gesamt. Augenheilk.," 2. Aufl., Bd 7a(2), pp. 1076-1225, W.
    Engelmann, Leipzig.

Mizuno, K., and Nishida, S. (1967)   Electron microscopic studies
    of human retinitis pigmentosa, Part I.   *Amer. J. Ophthal.* 63:
    791.

Noell, W. K. (1965) Aspects of experimental and hereditary retinal
    degeneration, in "Biochemistry of the Retina" (C. N. Graymore,
    ed.), pp. 51-72, Academic Press, London.

Noell, W. K., and Albrecht, R. (1971)   Irreversible effects of
    visible light on the retina: Role of vitamin A. *Science* 172:
    76.

Noell, W. K., Walker, V. S., Kang, B. S., and Berman, S. (1966) Retinal damage by light in rats. *Invest. Ophthal.* 5:450.

Noell, W. K., Delmelle, M. C., and Albrecht, R. (1971) Vitamin A deficiency effect on retina: Dependence on light. *Science* 172:72.

Recreational Innovations Company (October, 1974) *Technical News*, Saline, Michigan 48176.

Sloan, L. L. (1939) Instruments and techniques for the clinical testing of light sense. *Arch. Ophthal.* 22:233.

Sloan, L. L. (1944) A quantitative test for measuring degree of red-green color deficiency. *Amer. J. Ophthal.* 27:941.

SOCIAL SERVICES FOR HEREDITARY DISEASES

William B. Waters* and Thomas S. Baldwin

North Carolina Division of Services for the Blind*
P. O. Box 2658
Raleigh, North Carolina 27602

University of North Carolina School of Social Work
Chapel Hill, North Carolina 27514

INTRODUCTION

First, let me express my sincere appreciation for the invitation to appear on the program today. It is very rewarding to see this distinguished group of medical researchers holding a conference devoted exclusively to a better understanding of retinitis pigmentosa.

While the title of my talk today is "Social Services for Hereditary Diseases," I would like to address the question of services available to all blind and visually impaired individuals. For the client with hereditary eye conditions, special emphasis would be given to certain of these services during different stages of his development. For example, through the Genetic Counseling Program at the University of North Carolina at Chapel Hill, services are available to parents with a history of hereditary visual disorders to assist them in the process of family planning. During the early years of life, special counseling is available to the parents of children who are found to have hereditary eye disorders.

Recognizing these special areas of emphasis for the client with hereditary disorders, I would like to organize my remarks to you today under the following three headings. First, I would like to discuss my philosophy concerning the need for a comprehensive service program for the blind and visually impaired. As members of the medical profession, you are well aware of the importance of the medical components of such a comprehensive program. You may not be as familiar with the needs of the client for nonmedical, social, rehabilitation, and employment services that are so important for adequate life adjustment. It is only through a comprehensive service program encompassing both medical and non-medical services that the client can achieve his optimal self-fulfillment. Second, I would like to discuss with you the impact of various programs on the blind and visually impaired population in North Carolina. I believe through looking at the impact of present programs you may gain a perspective on the extent to which the needs of the blind and visually impaired are being made. Finally, I would like to discuss areas in work for the blind that I feel should be given priority for the future.

PHILOSOPHY ON WORK WITH PEOPLE WHO ARE BLIND

My philosophy concerning blindness is that the blind person is an individual whose lack of vision can be a serious handicap unless he is taught techniques and given counseling to develop a positive attitude toward his blindness that will allow him to compensate for his loss of vision. The individual should be given all services necessary for him to function to his fullest potential. If such a service program is available, his ability to function with proper training will be determined by certain variables, (just as with a sighted person) including intelligence, aptitude, manual dexterity, emotional stability, physical characteristics, etc. Too often the individual who is blind is thought of by the public as a "blind man" rather than an individual with certain characteristics, such as high intelligence, overweight, redheaded, blind, tall, etc. A comprehensive program of work for the blind will include a program designed to educate the public as well as a program that will enable the individual who is blind to adapt to the sighted world in which he must live. The sighted world will not make extensive adaptations for him; he must be given the services to develop his skills and attitudes to make the world less alien to him.

I believe that a program of services for the blind should be comprehensive in nature and treat the whole individual, not just his vocational needs, his social needs, or his medical needs. These services should be integrated so that the client does not feel that he is receiving fragmented services.

A comprehensive program of services should include first a sight conservation and a prevention of blindness program. Fifty percent of blindness in the U.S.A. is preventable, and from an economic and psychological standpoint, we should not allow one person to lose his vision when it can be prevented. Therefore, we must have an educational program that makes citizens aware of the need for good eye care and provide this eye care to the medically indigent who cannot secure it by themselves.

The first step in an individual plan of services should be to restore the individual's vision to the greatest extent possible. If his vision cannot be restored to the point that he can function independently, then adjustment services should be given that will allow him to compensate for his loss of vision. This includes teaching him such communication skills as braille, typing, signature writing, and independent travel techniques. Also, an adjustment program should have a strong "demands of daily living" emphasis. This should include teaching the housewife to continue normal activities, such as taking care of her children, cooking, cleaning, etc., and the unpaid family worker to function to his highest level of independence in such skills as indicated above. The program should also include family counseling, especially for the parents of children who are born blind, and counseling for the individual who is losing his vision. This State emphasizes the position that the individual who has a progressive eye condition should be started in an adjustment program as soon as possible after his progressive loss of vision is detected. Such a program eliminates much of the trauma which a person goes through while he is losing his vision and is more economical since habilitation is less expensive than rehabilitation.

If a person desires, he should be given an opportunity to achieve further independence through vocational training and placement programs. The individual who is blind is capable, with proper training, of participation in normal work activities. His abilities to achieve in the vocational world will vary with his individual characteristics such as intelligence, manual dexterity, and mental hygiene.

Because of the philosophy that a person should be given an opportunity to reach his maximum potential from a social, vocational, and psychological standpoint, it is my belief that workshops for the blind, such as the Lions Industries for the Blind in Durham, are a necessity. This philosophy is different from the philosophy of several states because generally, workshop employment is considered as sheltered employment. I believe that the individual who is blind and has additional handicaps such as mental retardation, should be allowed to produce, even though he cannot produce at a sufficient level to compete in industry. Well-managed workshops with well-trained personnel do not have profit incentives and can give employment to an individual who is blind and cannot meet the minimum standards required by industry; however, only after it is determined that he cannot compete in private industry. One of the reasons that North Carolina is a leader in rehabilitation in the nation is the fact that we have this resource. You will find that other states that are leaders in rehabilitation also have such resources.

A comprehensive service program should also have the ability to provide blind individuals with economic security through financial assistance. These money payments should be available to individuals who cannot, because of some factor such as age, earn their own livelihood.

It is also my feeling that more and more comprehensive adjustment services should be taken to the community and that individuals should not be displaced if they are to receive these services. These services should be available for the elderly as well as for individuals who are entering a habilitation or rehabilitation program.

I also believe that a program of services for the blind should be developed with consumer participation. There are several organizations of and for the blind in this state. The Division of Services for the Blind has tried to involve these organizations and individuals outside of these organizations in program planning and program implementation. Our society not only has a responsibility to individuals who are blind, but also the blind have a responsibility to society. If the blind are to achieve first-class citizenship and accept responsibility, they must be given the opportunity to participate in the development of a service program and, in addition, the individual who is receiving services must have the opportunity to participate in the development of his plan of services. I think such a program is necessary if we, as blind individuals, are to begin to see ourselves more and more as individuals who can contribute to society rather than to receive from society and expect more and more services that a well-adjusted blind individual can provide for himself. In other words, I am talking about a program that can provide the blind individual with dignity and the ability to feel that he has achieved first-class citizenship.

THE IMPACT OF PRESENT PROGRAMS

The second part of my remarks deals with impact of present programs for the blind. In North Carolina, we keep a register of known legally blind individuals. We have approximately 12,500 individuals on this register at present. The National Model Reporting System Area on Blindness estimates an efficient register will identify between two-thirds and three-fourths of the blind people in the state. Based on this statement, there are between 16,560 and 18,630 legally blind individuals in North Carolina. The number on the register is fairly stable from year to year and does not fluctuate since each month we add an average of 110 and remove an average of 110 due to sight restorations and deaths. This number has been fairly constant over the last ten years.

Medical/Eye Care Program

The National Society for the Prevention of Blindness has established that one-half of all blindness is preventable. Our Medical/Eye Care Program is designed to provide eye care services for the indigent population to detect ocular defects and provide services to correct these defects if possible. In the last fiscal year, we provided services to 43,358 citizens. This program restored vision to some degree to 23,506 citizens and prevented blindness in 19,851 citizens.

Social Services Program

This program provided services necessary for clients to remain self-sufficient. This program served 13,705 individuals in the last fiscal year, approximately 8,000 of whom were legally blind. The other individuals had ocular defects and felt they needed counseling to cope with the problems that this loss of vision was causing them.

Rehabilitation Program

This program is designed to provide services to the blind and visually impaired citizens to provide them with the opportunity to enter employment, or in the case of a housewife or unpaid family worker, relieve another member of the household in order that that member of the family might enter employment. In the last fiscal year, we rehabilitated into employment in productive work activities 1,150 blind and visually impaired citizens.

Concession Stand and Self-Employment Programs

Through these programs we provide employment opportunities to clients for whom opportunities are not available in the competitive labor market. The Concession Stand Program provided opportunities for 115 legally blind individuals to use their managerial talents in operating a concession stand. In addition, the Self-Employment Program provided employment opportunities for 175 clients who, through choice or necessity, remained at their own homes. These clients manufactured craft merchandise in their homes, thereby remaining productive members of the work force.

FUTURE DIRECTIONS IN SERVICES FOR THE BLIND

The third area that I would like to emphasize deals with the economic criteria for certain services. In particular, I feel that it is the responsibility of the State and Federal Governments to insure that all indigent citizens of our society have adequate medical eye care services. At present, it is my opinion that this is not the case. For example, in North Carolina we can now certify a family of four for eye care services if the family's earnings do not exceed $3,600. It is hard to imagine that a family of four with an income of $4,000, $5,000 or even $6,000 would be in a position to provide adequate medical eye care services for the family since the basic needs of food and shelter could not be met with that level of income. It is essential that we as a society must be more liberal in providing this important medical service to our indigent citizens. In addition, we should be in a position to provide all of our blind citizens with adjustment services such as braille, typing, mobility, and demands of daily living. In North Carolina there are 2,700 individuals, many of whom are elderly, who require these adjustment services each year and who are not enrolled in an intensive adjustment program. It is essential that these clients be provided with the training necessary to help them compensate for the loss of vision.

Another major area of need is for provision of comprehensive services to the visually impaired children in our schools (grades K - 12). There are many students in our school system with visual acuity of 20/70 or less who are not provided a good education today because they have not learned adequate adjustment techniques and do not have the equipment necessary to study as a visually impaired person.

We must also give attention to the development of hardware to assist the blind or visually impaired client in becoming more independent. In the past few years technology has had many break-throughs in developing instruments to assist the blind and visually impaired. For example, the optacon has been developed and enables a person who is blind to read print. Several other instruments with great potential in assisting the blind person to live a more normal life have been developed. However, the cost associated with these instruments is, at present, quite high and out of reach of most blind clients. Provision must be made to make these instruments widely available to those who need them.

Architectural barriers is another major area which must be emphasized. The primary emphasis in the removal of architectural barriers has been to individuals confined to a wheelchair. Emphasis on the removal of architectural barriers for those who are blind or partially sighted has not been studied and implemented. Architectural barriers include objects or projections in buildings and hallways that are about head high. In addition, deliberate effort should be made to help the partially sighted individual to identify steps, curbing, and other important obstacles to mobility.

Another major area of need is in research devoted to blindness. At present, the only significant area of research on blindness deals with medical aspects. While this represents an area that deserves major emphasis, there needs to be companion research efforts dealing with the adjustment of the client who has already lost his vision. Little is being done currently on the best ways of teaching the blind such skills as mobility, job modification for performance by the blind, and psychological and sociological factors which serve as barriers to the self-fulfillment of the blind person.

The development of professional personnel is an additional area that must be addressed if we are to provide the blind and visually impaired with adequate services to assist them in overcoming their handicap. It is essential that professional level programs in social and rehabilitation services be developed and that they address the special needs of the blind. At present, students can complete a Masters Degree Program in Social Work or Rehabilitation Counseling with virtually no attention to the special needs that confront the blind or visually impaired client. If graduates of these programs are to be expected to assist the blind client to make an optimal adjustment, it is essential that the universities in this country develop programs that will provide their graduates with the skills necessary in this area.

Another area that we need to pursue in work for the blind is a closer working relationship among the various professions. The trauma associated with the impending loss of vision causes psychological problems with which the client is often poorly equipped to deal. Oftentimes in progressive conditions, for which there is no known cure, the client denies the gradual loss of his vision and ultimate blindness. Until medical research can overcome the loss of vision from such disorders as retinitis pigmentosa, close working relationships between ophthalmologists, social workers, and rehabilitation counselors can help the client accept his loss of vision and make the necessary adjustments.

In closing, I would like to emphasize that we have come a long way in providing social services for the blind and visually impaired in less than the decade that I have been involved in work for the blind. Nevertheless, much remains to be done in terms of the numbers of clients served as well as the quality of services if our programs for people who are blind are to have their maximum effectiveness.

I have enjoyed meeting with you today and feel that this two-day program devoted to retinitis pigmentosa represents another milestone in the advancement of work for the blind.

DISCUSSION OF THE PAPER

DR. WOLBARSHT: Do you think it would be possible to think of
programs of visually handicapped (I am not necessarily referring
to retinitis pigmentosa, but other progressive diseases in which
we might try some more experimental approaches with people who are
willing to try them on either things to conserve what vision is
left, or to optimize the use of the vision that they do have left.
I mean, I know that it is a program in your program-oriented group
and the question is, then, is this something that you can conceive
of as part of a program?

DR. BALDWIN: Yes, Mike. This is one problem. We as an
agency have tried. I have been working on different state agencies
for seven or eight years and one of the first things that I was
involved in was trying to develop a research component--trying to
get the legislature to give us funds to do some of the kinds of
things that you are talking about. We haven't been successful so
far. It doesn't look as though we will be successful for the next
few years with the economy as it is, but we are able to do, with
program money, some of the things that you are talking about. I
think that it is entirely possible that it could be done.

PHOTIC INJURY TO THE HUMAN RETINA

M. O. M. Tso

Ophthalmic Pathology Division
Armed Forces Institute of Pathology
Washington, DC   20306

(Summary by M. L. Wolbarsht from conference recording)

Dr. Noell has presented several accounts of the damaging effect to the photoreceptor cells by light in rats with hereditary retinal dystrophy, as well as some other types of rats with higher intensities of light.   Additional material is presented here from human retinas to extend this model of damage by light to the retina.   However, a bit of caution is necessary as there are basic physiologic and pathologic differences between the photoreceptor cells of rats and primates such as rhesus monkeys and man.   Kuwabara has already noted that in rats the pigment epithelium was necessary for the regeneration of photoreceptor lamellas after photic injury, and if the pigment epithelium is severely damaged, the photoreceptor cells do not survive.   However, in experiments on monkeys exposed to light from either an argon laser or indirect ophthalmoscope, we showed the contrary.   A rhesus monkey exposed to an indirect ophthalmoscope light for one hour will develop degeneration of the photoreceptor elements, as well as necrosis of pigment epithelial cells.   The retinal pigment epithelial cells, however, will proliferate and spread into the necrotic region. However, the new cells do not contain melanin granules and are usually recognized as depigmented.   But the photoreceptor elements, including the rods and a layer of cones, are completely regenerated and there are no lost photoreceptor nuclei either.   It can also be noted in patients who have severe degeneration of the retinal pigment epithelium that photoreceptor cells overlying the degenerated retinal pigment epithelium do not regenerate immediately.

We have reviewed all of the cases of unusual exposure to sunlight and tried to connect this long term exposure to sunlight, or sun staring, with eclipse blindness in order to document any

functional loss or pathology.   Lifeguards in Atlantic City show a
short term depression in photopic sensitivity as well as a long
term loss of scotopic vision.   Pilots who have flown toward the sun
in order to avoid pursuit, as some did in World War II, have had
temporary loss of vision.   But in all of these cases the environment and other factors were constructed retrospectively.   The state
of the fovea before the exposure and the visual acuity, etc. were
not documented.   We have a series of three cases with malignant
melanomas who stared at the sun before the enucleation.   In the
first case, the only ophthalmological finding after sun gazing for
one hour was an increase in recovery from photo stress as measured
by the Henkin scotometer by a factor of three, from 55 seconds to
155 seconds.   Fluorescein angiography showed a distinct leakage of
fluorescein near the fovea.   Histological examination showed a
discrete lesion of 170 microns right in the middle of the fovea
and the rest of the retina appears normal.   However, the lesion
did not seem to disturb the patient's visual acuity (20/15).   The
second patient, who had had a previous slight vitreous hemorrhage,
showed approximately the same thing.   The third patient showed a
drop of visual acuity from 20/20 to 20/25.   Also, after an hour of
exposure to the sun, a definite central scotoma could be detected
by the Amsler Grid test.   Fluorescein angiography showed leakage
near the fovea about the size of the sun and histological examination showed a much larger lesion (350 microns) than the previous
two.   The third case had a dilated pupil, while the first two had
small pupils.   There were other marked changes upon histological
examination.   There was a shallow detachment of the photoreceptor
elements from the pigment epithelium, a marked sloughing of the
underlying pigment epithelium, with even some indications that
the pigment epithelial cells at the edge of the lesion were flattened and had started to grow to cover Bruch's membrane.   It has
already been mentioned that there were yellow spots seen ophthalmoscopically, probably due to the bolus detachment of the pigment
epithelium.   In all three patients, electron microscopy showed
dense bodies in the inner segment of photoreceptor cells.   There
are aggregates of lamellae.   We have never seen these in the normal
human fovea and they seem to be degenerative changes.   The outer
segments show particular and tubular degeneration and the pigment
epithelium shows loss of the apical melanin granules.   The remaining melanin granules were covered by a layer of lipoprotein-like
material.   The question comes that most sun gazers suffer severe
visual loss, yet the patients that we have observed suffered very
little.   This can be attributed to possible individual variations
between different people, and secondly that all histological examinations were within two to three days after exposure.

The fourth patient sun gazed for half an hour with a dilated
pupil and complained of being uncomfortable while sun gazing.   The
enucleation was performed ten days after sun gazing.   Funduscopic

examination immediately before enucleation showed a clearly visible
yellow area, a discrete lesion showing a central pigmented area
surrounded by the pigment epithelium. Fluorescein angiography at
that time, however, no longer showed the leakage which was present
two days after the exposure. Histological examination showed
many degenerated photoreceptor elements and loss of photoreceptor
nuclei. Macrophages appear to be very active, chewing up all of
the debris. The pigment epithelial cells have relined themselves
over the bare Bruch's membrane.

We learn from this that the human eye may be damaged by light
although the patient may initially be totally unaware of damage.
Secondly, there are probably great variations of susceptibility of
the retina of different people to photic injuries. Thirdly, the
damage resulting in the death of photoreceptor cells occurs several
days following injury. None of the patients morphologically show
the evidence of coagulation of protein either in the pigment epithelial cells or in the outer segments. The light damages these
photoreceptor cells in human patients in a way which causes only
minimal damage initially, but starts a degenerative process which
progresses continuously until the death of the photoreceptor cells,
with resulting blindness in that area. This does not seem to be
thermal coagulation, but the exact nature of the process is still
under investigation.

DISCUSSION OF THE PAPER

DR. LAVAIL: Could perhaps the variability be due to the
length of time that the person gazes? You mentioned one hour or
half an hour, in the case of that person, but the person who is
communing with God probably did so for a longer time. I wonder if
length of time would have anything to do with it or degree of pigmentation?

DR. TSO: Let me first say that the solar radiance varies with
the season and these four patients were collected over a period of
three years. So the solar radiance varies quite a bit at different
times. All of them sun gazed between 12 o'clock and 3 o'clock, and
I can tell any of you who want to know the exact solar radiance in
each case. We had a previous study using photocoagulation with a
xenon arc on a series of patients and we found that patients who
had the darker pigmentation in the pigment epithelium required less
energy to produce a similar amount of pathologic damage to the
retina. That manuscript is currently being prepared. But we do
suspect that the pigmentation of the fundi is a factor involved.

DR. LAVAIL. That is just the reverse of what I was driving at, actually. I have placed rats, which are supposed to be elegantly sensitive to the effects of constant light and are albinos or pink-eyed animals, litter mates in fact, and almost all of the photoreceptors are gone by 20-30 days in the pink-eyed animals. I can expose the pigmented animals for months and see maybe just a tiny loss of cells. Now, that is under a moderate amount of ambient light.

DR. LATIES: There are two ways to absorb light. There is light absorption by rhodopsin and light absorption by melanin. One system depends on one, most likely, and the other on the other.

DR. BERGSMA: Also, this is rather concentrated focal light and I presume that Matt (LaVail) is dealing with fairly high intensities of diffuse light.

DR. LAVAIL: Yes. Not even terribly high.